STRESS AND HEALTH

THE SERIES IN HEALTH PSYCHOLOGY AND BEHAVIORAL MEDICINE

Editor-in-Chief
Charles D. Spielberger

Byrne, Rosenman Anxiety and the Heart
Chesney, Rosenman Anger and Hostility in Cardiovascular and Behavioral Disorders
Crandall, Perrewe Occupational Stress: A Handbook
Elias, Marshall Cardiovascular Disease and Behavior
Forgays, Sosnowski, Wrzesniewski Anxiety: Recent Developments in Cognitive, Psychophysiological and Health Research
Gilbert Smoking, Personality, and Emotion
Hackfort, Spielberger Anxiety in Sports: An International Perspective
Hobfoll The Ecology of Stress
Johnson, Gentry, Julius Personality, Elevated Blood Pressure, and Essential Hypertension
Lamal Behavioral Analysis of Societies and Cultural Practices
Lonetto, Templer Death Anxiety
Morgan, Goldston Exercise and Mental Health
Morgan, William Physical Activity and Mental Health
Pancheri, Zichella Biorhythms and Stress in the Physiopathology of Reproduction
Sartorius et al. Anxiety: Psychobiological and Clinical Perspectives
Seligson, Peterson AIDS Prevention and Treatment: Hope, Humor, and Healing
Svebak, Apter Stress and Health: A Reversal Theory Perspective

STRESS AND HEALTH:
A Reversal Theory Perspective

Edited by
Sven Svebak
University of Trondheim
Trondheim, Norway

Michael J. Apter
Georgetown University
Washington, DC

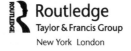
Routledge
Taylor & Francis Group
New York London

STRESS AND HEALTH: A Reversal Theory Perspective

Published 1997 by Routledge
52 Vanderbilt Avenue, New York, NY 10017
2 Park Square, Milton Park, Abingdon, Oxon OX14 4RN

Routledge is an imprint of the Taylor & Francis Group, an informa business

This book was set in Times Roman. The editors were Kathie Baker and Holly Seltzer. Cover design by Michelle Fleitz.

A CIP catalog record for this book is available from the British Library.

Library of Congress Cataloging-in-Publication Data

Stress and health: a reversal theory perspective/edited by Sven
  Svebak and Michael J. Apter.
    p. cm.—(Series in health psychology and behavioral
  medicine, ISSN 8756-467X)
    Includes bibliographical references.

    1. Clinical health psychology. 2. Stress (Psychology).
  3. Reversal theory (Psychology). 4. Medicine, Psychosomatic.
  I. Svebak, Sven. II. Apter, Michael J. III. Series.
  R726.7.S765 1997
  155.9'042-dc20   96-21820
                                                                        CIP

ISBN 13: 978-1-56032-473-7 (hbk)
ISBN 13: 978-1-56032-474-4 (pbk)
ISSN 8756-467X

Dedication

To Dagny Svebak, who coped with personal bereavement from childhood through her final year of life by caring for others, putting faith in God, and welcoming humor.—S.S.

To Vera Apter Smith, whose enthusiasm for life, openness to new experience, and concern for others continues to be an inspiration to her family and friends. —M.J.A.

Contents

Contributors

MICHAEL J. APTER, Psychology Department, Georgetown University, Washington, DC 20057, USA

ROBERT BATLER, Department of Psychology, Northwestern University, 2029 Sheridan Road, Evanston, Illinois 60208-2710, USA

EVELYN BROOKS, School of Nursing, University of Kansas Medical Center, 3901 Rainbow Boulevard, Kansas City, Kansas 66160-7502, USA

EDVIN BRU, The College of Rogaland, Stavanger, Norway

MARY R. COOK, Biobehavioral Sciences Section, Midwest Research Institute, 425 Volker Boulevard, Kansas City, Missouri 64110-2299, USA

DAVID FONTANA, Department of Education, University of Wales, College of Cardiff, Cardiff CF1 3YG, United Kingdom

KURT P. FREY, Psychology Department, Yale University, New Haven, Connecticut 06520, USA

MARY M. GERKOVICH, Biobehavioral Sciences Section, Midwest Research Institute, 425 Volker Boulevard, Kansas City, Missouri 64110-2299, USA

JOHN H. KERR, Institute of Health and Sport Sciences, University of Tsukuba, Tsukuba-shi, Ibaraki-ken 305, Japan

KATHRYN D. LAFRENIERE, Psychology Department, University of Windsor, 401 Sunset, Windsor, Ontario, Canada N9B 3P4

ANTONIA C. LYONS, Department of Psychology, Massey University, Palmerston North, New Zealand

ROD A. MARTIN, Psychology Department, University of Western Ontario, London, Ontario, Canada N6A 5C2

REIDAR MYKLETUN, The Norwegian School of Hotel Management, Stavanger, Norway

KATHLEEN A. O'CONNELL, School of Nursing, University of Kansas Medical Center, 3901 Rainbow Boulevard, Kansas City, Kansas 66160-7502, USA

JOHN SPICER, Department of Psychology, Massey University, Palmerston North, New Zealand

NAOMI SPIRN, Psychology Department, Northwestern University, 2029 Sheridan Road, Evanston, Illinois 60208-2710, USA

SVEN SVEBAK, Division of Behavioral Medicine, University of Trondheim, The Cancer Building, 5th floor, N-7006 Trondheim, Norway

LUCILIA VALENTE, Department of Child Education, University of Minho, Braga, Portugal

Preface

Why should the researcher working in such areas as behavioral medicine, the psychobiology of stress, somatic psychology, nursing research, or the study of addiction be interested in reversal theory? The simple answer is that reversal theory provides a way of looking at entrenched problems in these areas that is radically different from that of other approaches and that it is a theory for which there is an increasing amount of empirical support. It seems to us therefore that the theory merits the open-minded attention of serious researchers. How far it will eventually become assimilated into such fields as stress research and behavioral medicine is a matter for the future to decide. Many workers in these, and related, fields, however, have already found that it provides insights that are not obtainable elsewhere and that it opens up exciting new vistas for both research and application.

In the light of this, the aim of this book is to introduce reversal theory to those medical, psychological, and psychophysiological researchers who are not familiar with it, to show the kind of research it generates, and to provide a platform for those already doing research from the reversal theory perspective to communicate some of their main findings to others in their fields. It should also be of interest to those who have to deal with real, everyday problems of stress, addiction, and unhealthy behaviors of a variety of kinds.

In the first chapter, Kurt Frey sets the scene by providing an outline of reversal theory as a whole. This outline emphasizes the theory's generality, a generality that is unusual in these days of increasing specialization. As the reader will discover, stress and health form only a part of the scope of a broader theory that looks at all facets of motivation, emotion, and personality. (In fact, among other topics that it deals with in a systematic and integrative fashion are various types of neurosis and personality disorders, family relations, aesthetic experience, religious ritual, humor, violence, creativity, sexual behavior, sports performance, juvenile delinquency, risk-taking, and organizational development.) This chapter also brings out clearly the phenomenological grounding of the theory in the experience of everyday life. A feature of the chapter that those new to reversal theory will find helpful is a table and figure that summarize some of the characteristics of the metamotivational states identified in the theory; the reader may find this useful to refer back to as needed in reading later chapters.

The second chapter, by Apter, acts as a kind of bridge to the rest of the book, as it narrows and directs the concepts introduced in the first chapter into the focal interests of the book while still remaining general enough to provide a conceptual framework for all the chapters that follow. In other words, it takes such reversal theory concepts as metamotivational mode (or state), reversal, and metamotivational dominance, introduced in the first chapter, and shows how they can be applied systematically to the study of those problems that emerge where medicine and psychology overlap. The chapter also introduces and develops the important distinction between tension-stress and effort-stress.

In briefly reviewing the contents of the succeeding chapters, the use of technical terms from reversal theory is unavoidable. These terms and concepts are explained in the first two chapters. The five chapters that follow the introductory chapters make up a section of the book that deals with the effects of stress. First of all, Chapter 3 by Lafreniere provides evidence from a questionnaire study to support the reversal theory contention that telic dominance is a crucial mediator of the way in which stress is experienced. She also describes some intriguing gender effects that interact with telic dominance. Chapter 4 by Svebak examines the effects of stress on academic performance. His studies reveal a pattern in which stressors give rise to tension-stress, which in turn, as predicted by reversal theory, tends to give rise to effort-stress. The most successful students are those in whom effort-stress is highest, and these students not only achieve the best scores on the examination they have to take but are also those who are most successful at reducing their levels of tension-stress; their effortful exertions therefore have a double payoff in terms of both performance outcome and psychological state. In Chapter 5 by Svebak, Mykletun, and Bru, the effects of stress are again examined, but this time in terms of somatic consequences, specifically back pain. This work shows that the tension-stress that arises in different metamotivational modes has different effects on back pain. The main finding is that tension-stress that arises in the metamotivational mode known as the sympathy mode is associated with neck and shoulder pain. In Chapter 6, which also looks at somatic effects, various studies are reviewed by Martin and Svebak that clearly show that there are different patterns of response to stressful events in telic- and paratelic-dominant individuals. These differences are observable in terms of muscle tension for active and passive musculature, cardiovascular activation, and immunoglobulin A and cortisol secretion; an implication is that they put telic- and paratelic-dominant individuals at risk for different health problems. In the final chapter in this section, Spicer and Lyons in Chapter 7 explore the relation of telic and paratelic state and dominance to diastolic blood pressure reactivity. Interestingly, they find that the greatest reactivity occurs when telic-dominant students are in the paratelic state (and report feeling anxious). This opens a whole new area for future exploration (and one touched on also by Lafreniere in Chapter 3), namely the phenomenon that Spicer and Lyons call *mode-dominance misfit*. Taken together, these chapters show both that the tension-stress–effort-stress distinction is a useful one and that the modes and dominances identified in reversal theory are crucial to a full understanding of the experiential and biological effects of stress.

The following section of the book moves on to an area where a substantial amount of reversal theory research has been carried out, namely that of the physiology and psychology of smoking and attempts to quit this form of addiction. In Chapter 8, O'Connell, Gerkovich, and Cook start by reviewing some of their important previous research. The bulk of the chapter, however, reports on new research in which the authors include in their design, for the first time, measures of all four pairs of metamotivational states. In doing this they find that they are able, to an impressive extent, to predict whether a person who is attempting to quit smoking will lapse or resist in a tempting situation. In Chapter 9, the same team (Cook, Gerkovich, and O'Connell) study the physiological effects of smoking by means of electroencephalograph recordings. In doing so, among other things, they throw light on the well-known paradox that people seem to smoke at some times to stimulate themselves and at other times to become more relaxed. One of the key results that emerges from a complex data set is that, in terms of spectral analysis, telic-dominant people (and people in the telic state) smoke in such a way as to decrease arousal, whereas paratelic-dominant people (and people in the paratelic state) smoke in such a way as to increase it. There is much more in this chapter, however, which also reports on contingent negative variation and event-related-potential data in relation to both telic dominance and telic–paratelic state, showing a number of relationships. This study is an important one, as it is the first psychophysiological study of smoking using reversal theory concepts, and the results are encouraging for future research.

The next principal section of the book turns to a very different topic: risk-taking behavior. Apter has hypothesized that one major reason why some people take gratuitous, and even foolhardy, risks is that intense excitement may be achieved by overcoming danger, as this can trigger a telic-to-paratelic reversal during the time that the arousal caused by danger is at its highest. Evidence consistent with this hypothesis is provided in Chapter 10 by Apter and Batler, which reports on a questionnaire study of sports parachutists. In Chapter 11, Gerkovich examines a type of dangerous behavior that is especially serious in the era of AIDS, the performance of unsafe sexual practices. She shows that reversal theory can provide unique insights into such potentially destructive and self-destructive patterns of behavior. In particular, she proposes a detailed model, incorporating reversal theory constructs, and describes some preliminary evidence related to this model.

The final section of the book takes a positive orientation by looking at health-promoting behaviors and the factors that facilitate or inhibit them. In Chapter 12, Apter and Spirn report on a questionnaire study of volunteer blood donors and discover that although the altruistic motive (alloic sympathy) is, as one would expect, the strongest and most widespread one, nevertheless the motives related to all the metamotivational states are involved to different degrees with different donors. A practical implication is that calls for donors should appeal to more than the altruistic motive alone. In Chapter 13, O'Connell and Brooks ask an interesting question: What are the psychological similarities and differences between resisting urges to carry out old unhealthy habits (such as eating high-fat foods) and adopting new healthy habits (such as exercising regularly)? Their results show that success in both of these tasks is associated with being in the telic and conformist states. Failure, however, is associated with different metamotivational states in the two kinds of task. The next two chapters look at two forms of "antidote" to stress. Chapter 14, by Svebak and Martin, reviews research that the authors have carried out demonstrating in different ways that the experience of humor (which in reversal theory terms is a form of paratelic high arousal) has a buffering function in relation to the effects of stress. In Chapter 15, Kerr argues convincingly that exercise and sport may play a part in promoting health in stressful environments, either through helping people to change their arousal to suitable levels or by triggering reversals. He refers to research of his own (in collaboration with Vlaswinkel) that demonstrates both of these kinds of effects of exercise.

One of the principal themes in both Chapters 14 and 15 is that in the paratelic state stressors, causing high arousal and otherwise experienced as threats and problems, can instead become desirable forms of interest and stimulation. Indeed, this is one of the unifying themes of the book as a whole, picked up in different ways in many of the chapters. If some activity or situation can induce the paratelic state, then what would otherwise be stressful becomes not only less unpleasant but positively pleasant. The implications of this are potentially enormous. The negative side, also picked up in several chapters, is that in the paratelic state one can become dangerously oblivious to objectively real threats to one's health or even survival. Furthermore, the telic state also has its essential psychological uses, and the healthy individual needs to spend adequate time in both the telic and paratelic states.

Chapter 16, by Fontana and Valente, rounds out the book by exploring stress in the workplace. This chapter puts what has gone before in a wider perspective, by emphasizing the social and organizational context of stress. Of particular interest here is the idea that what has been called "corporate climate" can also be understood in metamotivational terms and that there can be degrees of metamotivational match and mismatch between employees and the companies for which they work. The chapter also proposes some practical strategies, derived from reversal theory, for use in coping with workplace stress. These strategies are discussed particularly in the context of stress management workshops.

The reader will realize from the preceding paragraphs that this book brings to the field of stress and health studies a perspective that is both coherent and distinctive. In particular, it suggests that there is a level of analysis (the metamotivational level) and a type of change (metamotivational reversal) that have been largely overlooked in previous work but that are critical components of people's healthy and unhealthy behaviors and their reactions to stress. If this is true, then reversal theory points to a whole new area for future research. In this respect, it is hoped that this book will prove to be seminal.

It is, finally, our pleasure to be able to record our gratitude to Professor Charles D. Spielberger, editor of the series of which this book forms a part, for his support and encouragement of this project from its inception; to Elaine Pirrone, the commissioning editor at Taylor & Francis, for all her expert help and advice during the period of writing and later; and to Bernadette Capelle, the development editor at Taylor & Francis, for her perspicacity in preparing the manuscript for publication. We also are very grateful to Holly Seltzer, production editor at Taylor & Francis, and Kathie Baker for their detailed editing.

Sven Svebak
Michael J. Apter

I

INTRODUCTION

1

About Reversal Theory

Kurt P. Frey

This chapter provides an introduction to reversal theory. Reversal theory is a general psychological theory that posits the existence of eight metamotivational states that combine in various ways to determine one's motives and experiences at a given moment in time. These states, occurring in pairs of opposites, are the telic and paratelic, conformist and negativistic, mastery and sympathy, and autic and alloic. Switches between opposite states are called reversals, which can occur as a result of contingencies, satiation, or frustration. Lability describes the reversal process, dominance moderates it, and structural disturbances can occur during it. Reversal theory is rooted in the phenomenological and structuralist traditions and describes people as inconsistent and self-contradictory and as wanting extreme, not moderate, experiences. Because people are so inherently psychologically diverse and unstable, healthy people are said to be motivationally versatile.

Reversal theory (Apter, 1982, 1989) is a general psychological theory that covers impressive theoretical territory and is applicable to all domains of human behavior and experience. More specifically, reversal theory is concerned with motivation, emotion, personality, and psychopathology. The theory has much to say about what people desire, their emotional makeup and vicissitudes, self-management, personality disturbances and clinical disorders, and interpersonal dynamics and relationships and about differences among people. The theory has provided penetrating insights into an ever-growing list of diverse topics: stress (the topic of this book), humor, sport, addictions, psychophysiology, depression, religious devotion, sexual behavior and dysfunction, work performance and satisfaction, hypnosis, delinquency, creativity, peak experiences, and so on. The list of international conferences, books, chapters, journal articles, and research projects inspired by the theory is also growing rapidly, if not exponentially. Besides Apter (1982, 1989), other good explications of reversal theory can be found in the following edited books on the theory: Apter, Fontana, and Murgatroyd (1985); Apter, Kerr, and Cowles (1988); Kerr and Apter (1990); and Kerr, Murgatroyd, and Apter (1993). Much empirical evidence—experimental, observational, psychometric, psychophysiological—can also be found in these books and elsewhere.

What, however, is reversal theory all about? What assumptions does it make? What concepts or processes does it refer to when explaining various psychological phenomena? How does it characterize human nature? What does it tell us that we don't already know? The purpose of this first chapter is to answer precisely these questions. The aim is not to survey the evidence that relates to the theory so much as to impart the basic ideas of the theory in a clear and immediately meaningful way, especially as these ideas relate to everyday life.

METAMOTIVATION

The centerpiece of reversal theory is a typology of distinct psychological states of mind. When people are in one of these states, they want a particular kind of experience. The states are said to be *meta*motivational because they determine what people want. And what people want is always in some way temporary. Motivation is fluid, not static. What people want right now may be very different from what they want an hour from now, a minute from now, or even a second from now. In different metamotivational states, people see the world— what they are doing, constraints on their behavior, their relationships with people and things, and the outcomes of these relationships—quite differently. Also, in different states people may actually think or process information quite differently. Moreover, in different states people experience distinctly different emotions. In various writings on reversal theory, these metamotivational states have also been referred to as *modes*, *ways of being*, or *selves* within the person.

So instead of describing what people generally desire, reversal theory describes the different things that people desire at different times, when they are in different states. In doing so, the theory focuses more on *intra*individual differences (differences within the person over time) than on *inter*individual differences (differences between people). You might try warming up to this idea of intraindividual differences by thinking about what you normally want and feel as you are climbing into a roller-coaster car versus a dentist's chair; about the kind of person you are when you are setting a New Year's resolution versus when, a month later, you are breaking that resolution; about how you feel when you are carefully listening to someone describe their problems at work versus how you feel when they are patiently listening to you describe your work-related problems; about your disposition when you are angrily exchanging malicious remarks with someone versus when, later on, you are sincerely apologizing to them; or about your attitude when you are out for a bike ride with a friend, immediately before she comments, "You're not in very good shape, are you?" and immediately afterward.

Reversal theory suggests that there are eight different metamotivational states: four pairs of opposite states. The idea that each state is opposite to another state is a key feature of the theory. Not only do people change from moment to moment (who would argue with such a commonsense notion?), but they change dramatically, going from one extreme to an opposite extreme. That is, they reverse from one state to its opposite (hence the name *reversal theory*). More is said about such reversals in a bit, but the point here is that each state is active when its opposite state is quiescent, and quiescent when its opposite state is active. Within each person there are very opposite desires, but these contradictory desires are spread out over time, so that they never actually confront each other.

Furthermore, the two states of a pair are said to be mutually exclusive and exhaustive: A person is always in one state or the other, never both at the same time or neither one. These two claims—that people cannot mix opposite states or be in some alternative third state—are consistent with the reversal theory claim that motivation is, at the psychological level, characterized by *bistability* (like a light switch or any device with two settings), not *unistability* (like a swinging pendulum that comes to a single stopping point). To say that people are bistable is to say that on particular psychological dimensions, there are two specific points (toward each of the extreme ends of the dimension) that are stable or optimal. Which point is optimal is determined by which metamotivational state is active and will change as prevailing states change. In this respect, reversal theory moves away from the simpler, and widespread, homeostatic accounts of motivation.

All of this amounts to the idea that one is, in any single moment, in four of the eight states, one state from each pair of states. Normally, however, one or two of the four active states will be more salient than the others. Salient states are those that have the greatest influence on behavior and experience. These four states, then, and especially the few that are most salient, determine people's temporary personalities—what they want, how they think, how they behave, the kinds of emotions they are likely to experience.

Indeed, reversal theory offers a novel definition of personality: Personality is the totality of one's metamotivational states and how these are articulated over time. Personality is not the way people are in a given moment; rather, personality is all that they are and the way that they change over time. One cannot grasp the dynamic nature of personality if one extracts the person from time.

Each of these eight states is now explored. Their principal characteristics are summarized in Table 1.

THE EIGHT STATES

Serious–Playful

The first pair of metamotivational states is made up of the *telic* and *paratelic* states. When in the telic state, the person is primarily goal-oriented. Attention is

Table 1   Principal Characteristics of the Four Pairs of Metamotivational States

TELIC	PARATELIC
Serious	Playful
Goal-oriented	Activity-oriented
Prefers planning ahead	Living for the moment
Anxiety-avoiding	Excitement-seeking
Desires progress–achievement	Desires fun and enjoyment
CONFORMIST	NEGATIVISTIC
Compliant	Rebellious
Wants to keep to rules	Wants to break rules
Conventional	Unconventional
Agreeable	Angry
Desires to fit in	Desires to be independent
MASTERY	SYMPATHY
Power-oriented	Care-oriented
Sees life as struggle	Sees life as cooperative
Tough-minded	Sensitive
Concerned with control	Concerned with kindness
Desires dominance	Desires affection
AUTIC	ALLOIC
Primary concern with self	Primary concern with others
Self-centered	Identifying with other(s)
Focus on own feelings	Focus on others' feelings

focused on some goal (flossing between hard-to-reach teeth, hailing a cab, proofreading a legal document for accuracy, passing a language proficiency test, reaching a sales quota, developing a vaccine for a deadly virus). The goal is what is important; the activities that enable one to reach the goal are much less important. In fact, if one could push some magical button that would automatically allow one to achieve that goal (the teeth are instantly flossed, the cab promptly hailed, the legal document thoroughly proofread, the language mastered, and the vaccine developed) without having to undergo the activities that lead to the goal, in the telic state one would gladly push that button.

   People in the telic state also tend to attach great importance to whatever goal they are currently pursuing, whether the goal is finding a low mortgage rate, making a good impression on a first date, or simply locating a bathroom in a desperate moment. Telic persons see whatever they are doing as having significant consequences (if not, then they are probably not in the telic state), and because telic persons are primarily goal-oriented, they eschew distractions and other sources of arousal. Although they want to be energized enough to pursue their goal, they do not want to be unnecessarily aroused or worked up. If the source of arousal seems frivolous or represents an obstacle or threat to goal achievement, it will produce in the person such negative emotions as anxiety and fear. Thus, persons in the telic state want to pursue goals (which are invariably deemed significant) in a calm and composed manner. (You might notice that a certain tension arises in the telic state, in the sense of wanting to remain calm and relaxed and yet wanting to have things be profound in their consequences.) Furthermore, to most effectively achieve goals, telic persons prefer to view events and circumstances in a realistic manner, becoming impatient with humor, artistry, or other forms of distortion. In general, being in the telic state means being serious.

Conversely, a person in the paratelic state is best described as being playful. The paratelic person is primarily activity-oriented, enjoying the very process of whatever they are doing or involved in—skipping stones on a lake, drinking lemonade at pool side, passionately kissing a lover during sexual foreplay, watching a television comedy, and so on. Although the person in the paratelic state may adopt some goal, the goal is somewhat arbitrary, simply serving as an excuse to engage in the activity. For example, wanting to feel the night air and gaze up at the stars, one decides to walk to the intersection of two country roads and back. Now if paratelic persons had the same magical button to push that would allow them to achieve their goal while obviating the activity (perhaps someone else could skip the stones on the lake, drink the lemonade, kiss the lover, or watch the comedy for them), they would balk at the idea. The difference between the telic and the paratelic states, then, has to do with whether the person is focused more on goals or activities, on ends or means.

Another important feature of being paratelic is not caring, not attaching much significance to what one is doing. In fact, one could say about paratelic persons that they could hardly care less. Of course they may be involved in a determined way in some strenuous activity such as playing a sport, but if they lose the playful quality of the game and start to really care, then they are no longer in the paratelic state. Furthermore, the person who is paratelic delights in arousing surprises and intense physical sensations. These—and various forms of humor, fiction, surrealism, and *cognitive synergy* (a reversal theory term for concepts or entities that possess dual identities, such as a child dressed up as an adult)—are found to be pleasantly arousing, exciting, and thrilling. Indeed, in the absence of intense physical sensations or stimulating peculiarities, the paratelic person will quickly succumb to boredom.

A final point to make about the paratelic state is that in it, emotions that are otherwise negative (in the telic state) can become positive. In fact, any emotion that involves high arousal will be enjoyed in the paratelic state. These emotions are referred to as *parapathic* emotions. For example, while watching a horror movie, what one feels is not true horror but rather something that one actually enjoys (this might be indicated by quotation marks, e.g., "horror"). Similarly, when one is paratelic, one often enjoy being "disgusted" (by a decaying carcass along the side of the road one stops to stare at), "grieved" (as when one rubbernecks at the scene of a tragic highway accident), "angry" (as when one plays the role of one who is angry), or "humiliated" (as when one endures a mock-whipping by a sex master in one's basement-turned-torture-chamber). When people do experience the more typical negative forms of particular emotions (e.g., feeling genuine disgust on stepping on a maggot-infested dead rabbit), it is clear that they are in the telic, not paratelic, state.

Compliant–Defiant

The second pair of opposite states consists of the *conformist* and *negativistic* states. Just as the telic and paratelic states have to do with emphasizing means versus ends, the conformist and negativistic states have to do with how one temporarily regards any restrictions on one's behavior. These restrictions may take the form of another person's expectations, norms more generally, rules, regulations, or traditions. The conformist person wants to conform to expectations and norms, respect and yield to rules and regulations, and live up to and cherish traditions—to become the pediatrician one's parents dreamed one would become, to behave as one should at a funeral, to buckle one's seat belt and drive the posted speed limit, to want everything to be just perfect in a grandiloquent church wedding. A person in the conformist state is compliant and respectful—the great defender of the status quo.

When in the negativistic state, in contrast, the person seeks freedom from all this. The negativistic person wants to defy others' expectations, mock norms, break rules and regulations, overthrow traditions—to wear outrageous clothes, tease a person about his or her weight, smash with a newspaper the fly that is buzzing around the apartment, swear profusely in the company of a divinity school friend or brag about one's sexual conquests to a celibate, spread a computer virus, or attempt to discredit some venerable scientific truth. In general terms, the person in the negativistic state gains pleasure from what is called in the theory *felt negativism*—the perception that one is to some degree violating rules.

One can begin to see how being in two states (one from each of two pairs of states) simultaneously can produce interesting blends of metamotivation. One can be *telic–conformist* (shopping for the right suit to interview in; working desperately to bring one's garden to bloom just like that of the neighbors across the street), *telic–negativistic* (banging on the car horn and making an obscene gesture to the maniac who has just run a stop sign; organizing a large-scale boycott of a company's products), *paratelic–conformist* (mindful of neighborhood rules and conduct while playing in a pick-up basketball game; taking delight in the use of chopsticks to devour a plate of moo goo gai pan at a Chinese restaurant), or *paratelic–negativistic* (facetiously mispronouncing someone's multisyllabic surname; engaging in taboo sex because it is taboo). Though norms and rules are not always the focus of people's attention, when they are, people are inclined to either comply with them or defy them, to go with the grain or against it.

Power-oriented–Affection-oriented

The third and fourth pairs of metamotivational states pertain to relationships—mostly people's relationships with other people, but also their relationships with inanimate objects (cars and computers), plants and animals (houseplants and pets), symbols and emblems (the American flag), or some objectified aspect of themselves (their toenails, their face, or their whole self in the form of *me*). In other words, these states concern different ways of experiencing what the theory refers to as *felt transactional outcome*—what one gains or loses in transactions with the world. They are therefore referred to in the theory as *transactional states*.

Specifically, the third pair of opposite states consists of the *mastery* and *sympathy* states. The person who is in the mastery-oriented state views a relationship as a power struggle and evaluates relationship outcomes in terms of who is winning and who is losing, who is strong and who is weak, who is dominating and who is submitting. In contrast, the person who is in the sympathy-oriented state views a relationship as a venue for affection and love and evaluates relationship outcomes in terms of intimacy, tenderness, nurturance, appreciation, and the like. Associated with all this, in the mastery state of mind one experiences pleasure in feeling hard and tough, irrespective of gaining or losing, and in the sympathy state one experiences pleasure in seeing oneself as sensitive and tender, again irrespective of outcome in terms of winning and losing.

Self-Oriented–Other-Oriented

Finally, then, the fourth pair of opposite states consists of the *autic* and *alloic* states. The person who is autic is primarily concerned with his or her own outcomes, whereas the person who is alloic is primarily concerned with the outcomes of the other (person, pet, computer, car) with whom he or she is relating. Combining the autic and alloic states with the mastery and sympathy states, one can see that one can be *autic–mastery-oriented* (bragging about your more lucrative or prestigious profession to an acquaintance at a high school reunion; attempting to navigate cyberspace), *autic–sympathy-oriented* (wishing that someone would visit you as you sit alone in your room in a nursing home; feeling deep gratitude at being thrown a surprise 60th birthday party), *alloic–mastery-oriented* (feeling overwhelming pride on being beaten by your son for the first time in a game of chess; marveling at the memory capacity or processing speed of your computer), or *alloic–sympathy-oriented* (giving a sensuous back massage to your lover; comforting a friend whose house has just burned to the ground).

Complicating matters slightly, people often identify with another person as they relate to someone or something else, wanting the person they are identifying with to be powerful in some way (if they are in the mastery state) or appreciated and loved in some way (if they are in the sympathy state). Thus, people often vicariously feel what others feel. They might identify with a protagonist in a novel, character in a film, a favorite basketball team during the playoffs, or a spouse who is home watching the kids. Such experiences, which do not involve a relationship between the self and some other but between some other and another other, represent a special case of the alloic state, referred to in reversal theory as the *pro-autic* state (Apter, 1988a).

Now when the other with whom the person is relating is his or her own self, as in the relationship between *I* and *me*, further metamotivational nuances occur. When *I* is attempting to dominate, control, or subjugate *me* (as when one pushes oneself to work long hours, exercise, go on a diet, or simply brush one's teeth or clip one's toenails), then one is simultaneously in the mastery state. When *I* is sympathizing with, appreciating, or nurturing *me* (as when one treats one's body to the hot tub, rests when one has the flu, compliments oneself as one models some newly bought lingerie in front of a mirror, or simply thinks better of oneself in moments of high self-esteem), then one is simultaneously in the sympathy state. Such experiences, which involve a relationship between the self as subject (*I*) and the self as object (*me*), represent a special case of the autic state, referred to in reversal theory as the *intra-autic* state. Being in the autic state but not in the intra-autic state is referred to simply as being *autocentric* (caring primarily about one's own outcomes in a relationship); being in the alloic state but not proautic is referred to simply as being *allocentric* (caring primarily about the outcomes of the other with whom one is relating; Apter, 1988a).

SIXTEEN PRIMARY EMOTIONS

For each of the metamotivational states there is both a preferred level and an actual level of each of various important experiential variables (how aroused one feels, how important or consequential things seem to be, how much one is abiding by versus breaking salient norms or rules, whether one is winning or losing in a relationship, and so on). The preferred level is determined by the metamotivational state itself (e.g., if one is telic, one prefers low arousal, but if one is paratelic one prefers high arousal). The actual level is determined by one's situation and perception of that situation. If the preferred and actual levels of a variable match, the person experiences positive emotions; if the preferred and actual levels of a variable do not match, the person experiences negative emotions. The degree to which such mismatching occurs is experienced as a kind of tension, a point that is taken up again in the next chapter.

Reversal theory claims that there are 16 primary emotions, corresponding directly to preferred and nonpreferred experiences in each of the eight metamotivational states. In the telic–conformist state one seeks to be relaxed or calm while trying to avoid feeling anxious. In the paratelic–conformist state one seeks to feel excited while trying to avoid feeling bored. Similarly, when one is telic–

negativistic one seeks to feel placid (not angry), whereas when one is paratelic–negativistic one seeks to feel mischievous or parapathically angry (not sullen). Moving to those states that have more to do with relationships, when one is autic and mastery-oriented one seeks to feel proud (not humiliated); when autic and sympathy-oriented, to feel grateful (not resentful); when alloic and mastery-oriented, to feel modest (not ashamed); and when alloic and sympathy-oriented, to feel virtuous (not guilty).

Figure 1 shows these relations among emotions in graphic form and makes it clear that there are two sets of general emotions involved. One set relates to

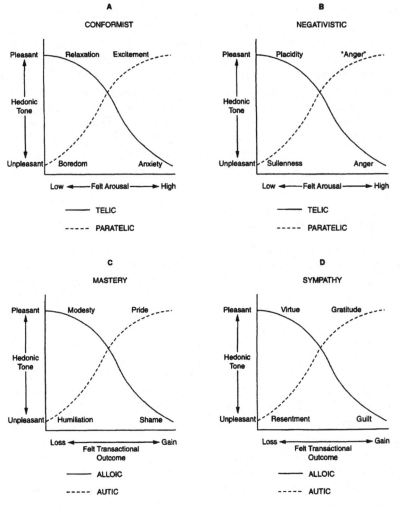

Figure 1 The relations between felt arousal and hedonic tone, or felt transactional outcome and hedonic tone, for each of the states in the four pairs of opposite metamotivational states.

felt arousal (remember that felt arousal is meant here to be how emotionally worked up the individual is); Figures 1A and 1B show the relationship between the telic and the paratelic states when these are combined with either the conformist or the negativistic states. The other set relates to felt transactional outcome (felt transactional outcome is meant here to be whether the individual experiences himself or herself to be gaining or losing as a result of the current transaction); Figures 1C and 1D show the relationship between the autic and alloic states when these are combined with either the mastery or the sympathy states. This means that at a given time the individual may experience emotions of both general kinds, that is, both an arousal-based emotion drawn from the relationships depicted in Figures 1A and 1B and a transactional emotion based on the relationships depicted in Figures 1C and 1D.

Although one could argue about the best emotion words to use, the more general argument is that all human emotions can in one way or another be assimilated to this basic structure of 16 primary emotions. Terror, for example, is an extreme form of anxiety. Envy (a form of humiliation) occurs when a person in the mastery state notices that another person (with whom they are in some way relating) has taken power, money, status, or privileges from someone or something else, whereas jealousy (a form of resentment) occurs when a person in the sympathy state notices that the other person has been given attention, affection, or love by someone else. (For more about reversal theory's account of emotions, see Apter, 1988b.)

THE REVERSAL PROCESS

As mentioned earlier, a reversal is a switch from one metamotivational state to the opposite metamotivational state. Often this involves a dramatic change in one's outlook and emotional experience. Think of click-clacking your way up to the highest peak of a roller-coaster, your clenched fists held defiantly overhead as you ready yourself for the precipitous rush downward, feeling intensely excited and euphoric when suddenly you hear what sounds like a wooden beam cracking or perhaps an axle breaking (only afterward do you realize that the sound emanates, quite naturally, from a mechanism in the track you are on). Unless you have a death wish or have eaten too much cotton candy to care, you reverse from the paratelic to the telic state, and the intense thrill you were feeling becomes acute fear. Although you continue to feel highly aroused, you now experience the high arousal very differently. Your personality has undergone a radical transformation.

In some ways, an even more interesting kind of reversal is one that occurs without any such obvious external impetus. One moment you are worried about having enough paper plates and plastic forks at a family reunion picnic; the next moment you no longer care about such things and decide to go tease your 40-year-old cousin about her 20-year-old fiancé. Evidently you have reversed from the telic–conformist state to the paratelic–negativistic state. Again you have experienced a profound personal transformation. Figure 1 shows graphically how a reversal involves experiencing the same level of a particular psychological variable quite differently from one moment to the next, and how dramatic this can be at the ends of the dimensions concerned, for example, from excitement to anxiety or from shame to pride. In other words, in the emotional space represented by these graphs, a reversal involves moving vertically from one curve to the other (or horizontally from one graph to the same position on the other graph, e.g., from anxiety to anger when there is a conformist-to-negativistic reversal).

Lability

The *lability* of a person—how readily or frequently he or she reverses back and forth between opposite states—varies at different periods. Sometimes reversals are likely to occur extremely frequently (as in the case of the rock climber, dangling on the face of a sheer cliff, reversing back and forth between intense anxiety and excitement many times in the course of even seconds). This phenomenon has been referred to, somewhat poetically, as *shimmering*. Other situations might find the person reversing between states a bit less frequently (as when one is talking on the telephone with a close confidant, dynamically moving from one topic to another, flip-flopping between states many times in the course of the conversation).

In other situations, or for other reasons, a person might reverse between states less frequently: After an hour or two of working on the garden, one now feels like diving into the swimming pool and luxuriating in the cool water, or after many hours of feeling angry at and defiant toward one's wife because of heartless comments she made, one finally reverses to the conformist and sympathy states, forgiving her and beginning to consider her hurt feelings. Certain extreme situations may find the person in the same states for longer periods of time: Imagine being in prison for the first time and feeling uncertain and telically anxious and fearful for many days on end. Although reversals probably occur every couple of hours, there are many reasons why they may occur more frequently or infrequently.

Mechanisms of Reversal

The concept of lability prompts a question that you may have already been asking: Why do people reverse between states? Basically, they do so for one (or some combination) of three reasons: *contingency, satiation,* and *frustration.*

Contingency   The first and most obvious reason why people reverse between states is that something occurs in the environment to instigate the reversal. Thus, the reversal is contingent on some external event. Indeed, as I wrote the last paragraph, I experienced a dramatic set of reversals. My 3-year-old son interrupted my typing to say that his orange juice (which I had poured for him earlier) tasted "yucky" and that he wanted me to pour him some more juice. In a primarily telic (and probably also conformist, autic, and mastery-oriented) frame of mind, I did not like being bothered with something so petty and did not respond kindly to his request. I immediately reversed to the negativistic state. He then further explained, "It tastes like water with soup and hair in it," a description that struck me as very funny and that caused me to reverse to the playful paratelic and kindly alloic and sympathy-oriented states. My personality immediately changed: I grabbed and hugged him, tickled him, talked with him, and poured him some fresh orange juice. That done, as I looked at the clock and considered how much writing I wanted to accomplish, I reversed back to previously active states and resumed my work.

Thus, reversals occur because things happen: One overhears a radio news announcer say that the stock market has plunged or that gratuitous murder and rape are occurring in some foreign country; one notices someone walking along in sexy attire; one senses the sarcasm of a condescending sales clerk; one realizes that one's words have caused someone to burst into tears; and so on. Now, to be sure, environmental events or contingencies do not always bring about reversals, and the same events may more or less incur reversals or incur different reversals in different people. However, the previously described episode with my son is a good example of the kind of internal changes that everyone experiences many times in the course of their daily lives. Though perhaps not profound to an observer, from a subjective viewpoint such changes in a person's temporary personality can be quite dramatic and profound.

Satiation　A second mechanism of reversal is that of satiation, which refers to the idea that, even in the absence of any environmental contingencies, the person will eventually undergo a reversal. One can only be serious, playful, defiant, compliant, power-oriented, affection-oriented, self-centered, or other-centered for so long before a reversal to the opposite state will spontaneously occur.

Think of lying down on the sofa to calm down and relax and then suddenly having the desire to call up a friend to go bowling. Think of attending a committee meeting and suddenly feeling the desire to say something provocative, sarcastic, or off-color. Think of having an intimate, affectionate conversation with someone and suddenly feeling like having a contest with them or going off somewhere to compete with them. Think of sitting sympathetically at the bedside of a relative with terminal cancer, when suddenly the desire to go have sex or out to a restaurant overtakes you. Satiation, then, is the idea that meta-motivational shifts eventually occur automatically. Just as there are important biological rhythms, there are important psychological (in this case, metamotivational) rhythms. One may not, however, be aware of such rhythms because they may be swamped by environmental events and contingency-produced reversals.

Frustration   A final mechanism of metamotivational reversal is that of frustration, which refers to the fact that when a person is in a particular state and goes without achieving the satisfactions of that state for too long, they may spontaneously reverse to the opposite state. Feeling that you want to care for others but not having any immediate way of doing so, you might reverse to the autic state. Feeling playful and frivolous but not having anything adequately stimulating to do, you might reverse to the telic state. Feeling sympathy-oriented but realizing that you are operating in a cutthroat environment, you might reverse to the mastery state. When one is not getting what one wants, eventually one spontaneously reverses to an opposite state of mind in which one is less likely to be so frustrated.

It should be mentioned that reversals do not occur because one has direct control over them. According to reversal theory, people cannot willfully reverse from one state to another. They can only indirectly control reversals and which states are active in a situation by engineering the contingencies that are likely to bring about reversals (as when one goes to the beach for the day, deliberately leaving all the trappings of work behind).

Dominance

Why is one event likely to bring about a particular reversal in one person and not another? Why does one person satiate more quickly than another? Why is one situation dissatisfying and frustrating for one person but not another? The answers to these questions lie, in part, in the concept of *dominance*, which suggests that each person spends relatively more time in one of the states than in its opposite. A person might, for example, be paratelic-dominant, spending more time in the paratelic state than most people. Conversely, one might be telic-dominant, spending more time in the telic state than the average person. Similarly, one is either conformist- or negativistic-dominant, mastery- or sympathy-dominant, and autic- or alloic-dominant. Each person has a bias (which might be learned or perhaps genetically programmed) for one or the other states in each of the four pairs of opposite states. These biases, and the extent of these biases, represent important interindividual differences (see Svebak & Murgatroyd, 1985, for illustrative examples of dominance).

The concept of dominance is a bit different than that of a trait. Possessing a particular trait—being an introvert or an extravert, for example—suggests that the characteristic is a stable, enduring aspect of one's personality. Dominance, however, simply suggests that the person spends more time in a particular state. To say that a person is, for example, mastery-dominant is not, however, to imply that he or she is always in the mastery state or that when a person is in the sympathy state, he or she is not as sympathy-oriented as the person who is sympathy-dominant. Dominance refers to the frequency or likelihood of being in a particular state without reference to the content of experience in that state. Presumably, there are more contingencies that reverse one into one's dominant than into one's nondominant state, and one satiates more slowly and is less easily frustrated in one's dominant state.

The concept of dominance offers a bit of balance to reversal theory. Although the theory emphasizes that people are inconsistent, the concept of dominance suggests that there are important consistencies behind their inconsistencies. Although intraindividual differences are profound and remarkable, interindividual differences are also important. The differences within one person over time are often more profound and remarkable than the differences between him or her and another, but the differences between them are also significant, at least from a theoretical perspective.

Structural Disturbances and Inappropriate Strategies

A person may experience a certain amount of inhibition when it comes to reversing from one state to its opposite, a case of *inhibited reversal*. For example, the person may continue to be telic even at parties or have difficulty reversing from a sympathetic mind-set to a tough, assertive, mastery-oriented mind-set. Alternatively, one may reverse too readily or, more to the point, inappropriately, a case of *inappropriate reversal*. One may too easily become flippant or jocular (paratelic) during a murder trial or self-absorbed (autic) while teaching a class of kindergartners. Inhibited and inappropriate reversals are called *structural disturbances* because something is amiss in the dynamic structure of one's metamotivation.

Another type of problem arises when the person uses inappropriate strategies when attempting to satisfy the desires of particular states. Strategies can be functionally inappropriate (the person engages in a behavior that is not effective in satisfying the desires of the active state), as when one goes camping to leave behind the cares of the world, only to turn every detail of the trip into a worry. Strategies can be temporally inappropriate (the person engages in a behavior that does satisfy the desires of the active state but that is dissatisfying to a state that is activated later or injurious to the person more generally), as when one spends a lot of time socializing with others while neglecting one's work duties. Finally, strategies can be socially inappropriate (the person engages in a behavior that is quite satisfying to his or her own state but that is very dissatisfying or injurious to other people), as when one drives on the freeway as if in a stock car race, creating havoc and danger for the more sedate, conscientious drivers (see Murgatroyd, 1987, for reversal theory's approach to psychotherapy).

THEORETICAL ROOTS AND HALLMARKS OF HUMAN NATURE

The final part of this chapter fills in some of the obvious gaps in the preceding characterization of reversal theory by describing the theoretical roots of the theory as well as what it suggests are the hallmarks of human nature.

Theoretical Roots

The theoretical roots of reversal theory are in the phenomenological and structuralist traditions (which is why the approach taken by the theory is called *structural phenomenology*). Reversal theory is phenomenological in the sense that it is concerned with subjective experience more than with objectively observable behavior. It is not that behavior is deemed unimportant, but rather that behavior cannot be fully understood without exploring the motivation that underlies it. There is not a one-to-one correspondence between motivation and behavior or between behavior and experience. Two individuals might engage in the same behavior but in different metamotivational states (resulting in different, even opposite, experiences), or the same individual might engage in the same behavior but in different metamotivational states at different times. It is for this reason that reversal theory prefers the term *action* over the term *behavior*, action being behavior plus subjective meaning. Thus, reversal theory takes an inside-out approach (starting with motivation and experience and then interpreting behavior in light of these), regarding any strict or dogmatic brand of behaviorism (which disregards motivation and experience as irrelevant epiphenomena of behavior) as a kind of methodological vandalism (Apter, 1989).

From the structuralist tradition (e.g., in the fields of anthropology and linguistics), reversal theory derives the idea that subjective experience is structured. The claim is not that the products of the human mind (such as myth, culinary, or linguistic systems) are structured (as in structural anthropology) or that the contents of the human mind are structured (as in Gestalt psychology), but that experience itself is structured. Behind all the various ups and downs and comings and goings of one's different motives and emotions are a fixed set of states. Particular aspects of experience are related (through polar opposition) to other aspects of experience. The structure of experience lies in the eight metamotivational states; the dynamic nature of this structure lies in the reversal process and articulation of states over time.

Thus, reversal theory represents the hybridization of two robust traditions in the social sciences, traditions that have heretofore repelled each other because they are relatively hard and soft, deterministic and indeterministic, respectively (Lachenicht, 1985).

Hallmarks of Human Nature

Reversal theory provides its students with an unambiguous, and rather iconoclastic, description of human nature. To begin with, reversal theory emphasizes that people are inconsistent and self-contradictory. People want very different experiences at different times: What a person wants right now may not be what he or she wanted an hour ago or what he or she will want an hour from now. People undergo radical transformations in their personalities during relatively short periods of time. As Marcel Proust put it, "All decisions are made in a state of mind that is not going to last." No wonder people have a hard time understanding themselves. No wonder that others have a hard time understanding them. What they are trying to understand is constantly changing. And with the environment constantly changing and people's selves constantly changing, it is no wonder that self-management is no easy task and that joy and satisfaction are elusive.

Furthermore, reversal theory suggests that people typically want extreme, not moderate, experiences. It was mentioned before that reversal theory claims that many important psychological variables are bistable. One wants either a lot of arousal or very little arousal. One wants things to be very important and consequential or trivial and meaningless. One wants to uphold laws and cherish rituals or break totally free of restraints. One wants to exchange sympathies or exchange blows. Now it may be that people sometimes opt for a moderate level of some variable out of necessity, such as when they prefer to be moderately aroused, even a bit anxious, in order to complete a task. Such instances, however, represent concessions and not what the person most essentially wants. *All things in moderation* may be true of what the person wants averaged over time, but it is never true of what the person really wants at any single moment in time.

Finally (and these various hallmarks of human nature are not completely distinct or comprehensive), the healthy person is characterized by instability, not stability. People are constantly changing, and they should be constantly changing. It is their nature (whether by design or the result of millennia of evolution) to be always fluctuating and shifting about. Should their changeability be forestalled, they are in trouble (of course, if they are too changeable or inappropriately changeable, then they are also in trouble). If healthy persons are at all stable, it is in their stable use of functionally, temporally, and socially appropriate strategies to satisfy state-determined desires and in their stable ability to exert indirect control over the reversal process and over which states are active in a situation in a fairly efficacious way. Although one tends to think of the healthy person as being psychologically stable, it is probably more true that such a person is dynamically unstable, albeit in a skillful, adroit way. Characterized by *psychodiversity* (possessing a rich diversity of motives that come and go in time), the healthy person exhibits *motivational versatility* (the ability to activate states that best match each situation and occasion).

REFERENCES

Apter, M. J. (1982). *The experience of motivation: The theory of psychological reversals.* London: Academic Press.

Apter, M. J. (1988a). Beyond the autocentric and the allocentric. In M. J. Apter, J. H. Kerr, & M. P. Cowles (Eds.), *Progress in reversal theory* (pp. 339–348). Amsterdam: Elsevier.

Apter, M. J. (1988b). Reversal theory as a theory of the emotions. In M. J. Apter, J. H. Kerr, & M. P. Cowles (Eds.), *Progress in reversal theory* (pp. 43–62). Amsterdam: Elsevier.

Apter, M. J. (1989). *Reversal theory: Motivation, emotion, and personality.* London: Routledge.

Apter, M. J., Fontana, D., & Murgatroyd, S. (Eds.). (1985). *Reversal theory: Applications and developments*. Cardiff, Wales: University College Cardiff Press.

Apter, M. J., Kerr, J. H., & Cowles, M. (Eds.). (1988). *Progress in reversal theory*. Amsterdam: North Holland.

Kerr, J. H., & Apter, M. J. (Eds.). (1990). *Adult play*. Amsterdam: Swets & Zeitlinger.

Kerr, J. H., Murgatroyd, S., & Apter, M. J. (Eds.). (1993). *Advances in reversal theory*. Amsterdam: Swets & Zeitlinger.

Lachenicht, L. (1985). Reversal theory: A synthesis of phenomenological and deterministic approaches to psychology. *Theoria, 64*, 1–29.

Murgatroyd, S. (1987). Reversal theory and psychotherapy: A review. *Counseling Psychology Quarterly, 3*, 371–381.

Svebak, S., & Murgatroyd, S. (1985). Metamotivational dominance: A multimethod validation of reversal theory constructs. *Journal of Personality and Social Psychology, 48*, 107–116.

2

Reversal Theory, Stress, and Health

Michael J. Apter

This chapter shows how the general concepts of reversal theory can be applied to the study of stress and of health-related behaviors. It does so in terms of five broad themes:

1. A major source of stress is tension, defined as a discrepancy between the preferred and actual level of a variable operated on by a metamotivational state.

2. When the paratelic state is operative, any strong emotion becomes pleasant, even a supposedly negative one, as the preferred level of arousal is high in this state; this is another way of saying that stress can be enjoyable.

3. Any attempt to reduce tension that requires effortful activity also constitutes a type of stress, and such effort-stress can be contrasted with tension-stress.

4. To understand either type of stress, either at the psychological or the psychobiological level, it is necessary to know which are the concomitant operative metamotivational states; the same is true in understanding unhealthy behaviors.

5. An understanding of healthy and unhealthy lifestyles also requires that one take into account the reversal process, which adds an element of instability at the metamotivational level.

As the reader who is unfamiliar with reversal theory will have discovered from Chapter 1, the theory is a rather general one that can be brought to bear on a diverse range of behaviors and experiences. Chapter 1 also presented some of the basic concepts of the theory and showed how they provide a distinctive and coherent approach to an understanding of motivation, emotion, personality, and other related psychological topics. The aim of this chapter is to take matters a step further by exploring the relevance of these concepts to the particular subject matter of this book, namely to the study of stress and of health-related behaviors. Later chapters document detailed studies in these areas. The intention here is to provide a systematic context for these studies by setting up a general framework, based on reversal theory, in which they can be placed. This is done in terms of five broadly related themes.

THE VARIETIES OF TENSION-STRESS

One of the central themes of Chapter 1 is that there is a set of states, referred to in the theory as metamotivational states, that a normal person will be expected to pass through on a reasonably frequent basis during the course of ordinary everyday activity. These states represent ways of being in the world, and they come in pairs of opposites so that each such way of being is opposed by a contrary one, with movement from one to the other constituting a reversal.

One aspect of these states is the emotions with which they are associated. More specifically, when they are combined in pairs, in the way described in the previous chapter, a distinctive range of emotions can be related to each such pairing (Apter, 1989, 1991a). As was shown in Figure 1, each range extends from a highly positive emotion to an opposite and highly negative emotion, with weaker versions of these emotions coming in between. Eight basic emotional dimensions, or polarities, emerge from the state combinations, each with its own particular range of emotions; this means that there are eight basic unpleasant emotions. These are, specifically, anxiety, boredom, anger, sullenness, humiliation, shame, resentment, and guilt. Each of these negative emotions has its own phenomenal quality, but they share something in common, namely a kind of unease or discomfort, a feeling of a need to change and to seek out the pleasant end of each dimension concerned. This unhappy, restless, and strained feeling can be referred to as tension.

The further away from the pleasant and therefore desirable end of a given dimension the individual experiences himself or herself as being, the greater the tension that will be felt; in other words, the greater the mismatch between the preferred value of the underlying variable (e.g., felt arousal) and the actual value of that variable, the greater the tension. The converse is that where the preferred and actual values are acceptably the same, so that there is matching rather than mismatching, there will be no tension and the person will feel at ease with the agreeable emotion that is being experienced. Reference to Figure 1 will make clear that tension in principle can be reduced in two ways, either by changing the value of the variable concerned or by reversing to the opposite metamotivational state. (Good examples of actions involving these alternatives can be found in Chapter 15 by Kerr.)

It should be clear, incidentally, that tension defined in this way is not to be equated with arousal. The simplest way of making this distinction evident is to point out that not only can high arousal be related to tension (as it is, e.g., in the case of anxiety), but low arousal can also represent tension (as occurs in the experience of boredom). Indeed, the tension may come from some source that in itself has nothing directly to do with arousal, either high or low, for example, the tension of resentment.

Now tension as defined here is clearly a form of stress. Whether one is talking about anxiety or anger or guilt, or some other negative emotion, one is referring to a disagreeable feeling that relates to an undesirable state of the world for the individual concerned. To put it another way, whatever the particular nature of the stressor—be it, for example, danger, frustration, defeat, or unfairness—the immediate psychological effect will be one or another of the basic forms of negative affect. These can all be referred to as forms of tension-stress (which is contrasted, below, with what is called effort-stress).

In the normal way of things, there may well be more than one form of tension at a given time; for example, the tension of anxiety and the tension of guilt may both be felt together. There would seem to be no reason in principle why one should not think of different co-occurring tensions as summating in some way, so that one can conceive of all the tensions in consciousness at a given time as coming together to produce an overall level of tension-stress at that time.

Finally here it should be noted that as far as any particular type of tension-stress is concerned (e.g., anxiety, resentment), there are all kinds of factors that may facilitate or inhibit that particular stress in a given individual. For instance, in a telic-dominant individual (someone who is frequently in the telic state), an innate tendency to be easily arousable will produce the frequent experience of tension-stress in the form of anxiety. In contrast, low arousability associated with telic dominance will tend to produce a low frequency of tension-stress. In the paratelic-dominant individual, matters will be quite the other way around, with a high frequency of tension-stress being associated with low innate arousability and a low frequency of tension-stress with high arousability. Data consistent with this have been reported by Lafreniere (1993). It is important to notice that this analysis depends on a distinction between arousability (how easily the individual is aroused) and arousal preference (what level of arousal the individual actually wants at a given time). This is an important distinction and one that tends to be overlooked or blurred in other theories of personality and emotion.

To take another example of the facilitation or inhibition of tension-stress, different organizations in which people work may provide more opportunities for the satisfaction of one state than of its opposite, so that the individual whose dominance works against the tendency of the organization may be expected to experience more tension-stress at work than someone for whom this is not the case. Fontana develops this theme in Chapter 16 of this book.

THE ENJOYMENT OF STRESS

If one takes stressors in the conventional sense as those things that cause bad emotions, such as threats that cause anxiety, failures that cause humiliation, and inequities that cause anger, then one can deduce something surprising from reversal theory. This is that under the right circumstances such stressors are not really stressors at all, but are highly desirable, sought out when lacking, and enjoyed when available.

"The right circumstances" means here when experienced in the presence of the paratelic state. The reason is that in the paratelic state all forms of high arousal, whatever their source, become hedonically positive and are experienced in some fashion as stimulating, exciting, or even thrilling. In other words, in the paratelic state all strong emotions are good, even supposedly bad ones—in this state the valence of all negative emotions is inverted. So it is now possible to enjoy the anxiety of a closely fought basketball game, the horror of a horror film, the thrill of driving too fast, the pathos of a Puccini opera, or the grief of a Shakespearean tragedy. In all these cases, the bad emotions have been converted, through the medium of the paratelic state, into pleasurable emotions. Such emotions are known in the theory as *parapathic* emotions. The trick of enjoying bad emotions, then, is to find some way of experiencing them parapathically. Indeed, much of human culture is about setting up conditions that encourage precisely this: sports fields, golf courses, casinos, theaters, cinemas, and so on. In this way people can experience such emotions as parapathic anxiety, parapathic anger, parapathic resentment, and the like. They can even do so in the comfort of their own homes, in front of the television set, for example, watching a soap opera.

The examples of television, cinema, and theater are a reminder that humor is another kind of pleasant strong emotion. In the terms defined here, humor is not technically a parapathic emotion because it does not have an unpleasant telic counterpart. It is, however, a special form of paratelic excitement (see Chapter 14 by Svebak and Martin).

One implication of all this is that a lack of stimulation, which could be described as a lack of stressors, can be as stressful as the presence of stressors. That is, in the paratelic state stressors—in the form of challenges, puzzles, risks, and so on—are needed, and needed as much as they are unwanted in the telic state, where they are experienced as threats, dissonances, and problems. Paradoxically, it is the absence of such problems rather than their presence that is dysphoric in the paratelic state. Such absence is experienced as tension in the form of boredom, and such tension-stress may be every bit as unpleasant in its own way as the tension-stress of anxiety or some other form of telic high-arousal emotion. (Indeed, de la Pena, 1983, has argued that boredom is a health problem that is every bit as serious as anxiety and has presented detailed evidence that it may even be implicated in the development of cancer.)

Consistent with this analysis of the enjoyment of stress-generated arousal, Martin and his colleagues in Canada (Martin, Kuiper, & Olinger, 1988; Martin, Kuiper, Olinger, & Dobbin, 1987) have shown that people who are paratelic-dominant— that is, who are often in the paratelic state—become disturbed by a lack of stressors in their lives, at least up to a certain level of stress, in comparison with telic-dominant people, who alone display what is commonly supposed to be true of everyone: They become more disturbed the more the stress they experience. Paratelic-dominant people, therefore, at least up to a certain level, thrive on stress and seek it out in their lives. That this desire for stress is true for them only up to a certain level is probably because beyond this point they switch into the telic state and start to display the telic pattern. This line of research is taken up again in Chapter 6 by Martin and Svebak.

Supposed stressors may also have their psychological satisfactions in relation to other metamotivational states. This is perhaps particularly true of the negativistic and the mastery states. In the negativistic state, the stress of confrontations, arguments, and disagreements may be exactly what is required to provide a focus for the negativism and an excuse to behave defiantly or badly. In the mastery state, the stress that derives from being faced by difficult problems may provide the occasion for the display of ability, expertise, and skill and the opportunity for eventually experiencing control and feelings of efficacy and power. So confrontations may be sought out by someone in the negativistic state, and problems may be sought out by someone in the mastery state.

The moral of all this is that things are not so straightforward as they might seem when it comes to defining stress. What is stressful to one person in one state (e.g., exercise, the topic of Chapter 15 by Kerr, or risky sexual situations, as discussed by Gerkovich in Chapter 11) may be not only not stressful but actually highly desirable to someone else, or to the same person in the opposite state at a different time. Human nature is more paradoxical—and much more interesting—than would appear to be the case from more traditional accounts in the human sciences in general and the literature on stress in particular.

TENSION-STRESS VERSUS EFFORT-STRESS

When people experience tension, what do they do about it? One possibility is to do nothing and put up with it. The other is to take some kind of action in order to attempt to change the situation that is bringing about the tension. Thus, if one is anxious, then one might simply endure the anxiety; alternatively, one might go out and do something about whatever is causing the anxiety, if this can be identified. If one is anxious that one is going to fail an examination, for instance, one can remain anxious and do nothing or work hard to deal with the course material and in this way remove the reason for the anxiety. There are all the intermediate possibilities represented by doing more work than one had been doing and in this way removing some, but only some, of the cause for anxiety.

The downside about taking effortful action is that the effort involved is itself stressful in some sense. That is, taking action and working at something in order to reduce a tension, whatever the form of the tension (anxiety, guilt, resentment, etc.), may also be said to represent a kind of stress or strain. Phenomenologically this is experienced as being determined, as putting oneself out, as trying hard, and so on. The key aspect of this experience is being effortful, and so this kind of stress can be described as effort-stress in order to contrast it with tension-stress.

This means that there are two intrinsically different forms of stress (Apter, 1991b; Apter & Svebak, 1989; Svebak, 1991a, 1991b). The first is about the experience of tension, about mismatching (in terms of certain key motivation variables like arousal level or felt transactional outcome), and about the subjective awareness of an unsatisfactory situation. The second is about trying to cope with that situation, about the experience of dealing with that tension, and about attempting to overcome the mismatch and bring the variable concerned into an acceptable range of values. (A measure of these two forms of stress, known as the Tension and Effort Stress Inventory, has been developed by Svebak [1991a, 1993] and is described in Chapter 5 by Svebak, Mykletun, and Bru.)

It has already been shown that what is an unpleasant emotion in one state becomes, following a reversal, a pleasant emotion in the opposite state. That is, level of tension and therefore hedonic tone inverts following a reversal. (The implications of this are discussed later in this chapter.) Does something similar happen to effort-stress? The answer seems to be yes, but only for the telic–paratelic pair. That is, what is a chore and work in the telic state (unpleasant effort-stress) becomes a challenge and fun in the paratelic state. In the paratelic state, people are willing to exert themselves (e.g., playing sport) and be joyfully exuberant. In other words, effort-stress is not really stressful in the sense of being unpleasant when the paratelic state is operative, in just the same way that an unpleasant strong emotion, like anger or guilt, is also not unpleasant but actually enjoyed in the paratelic state. In this sense, the paratelic state is paradoxical, turning much of everyday language upside down.

So the telic and paratelic states differ in the way in which they experience effortful activity, as well as in other ways. The need that paratelic-dominant people have for stressors as demonstrated in the work of Martin et al. (1987, 1988; discussed above) probably reflects this aspect of the two states as well as the different ways in which arousal is experienced by these states.

As either the telic or the paratelic state is always in operation, this aspect of effortful activity will color such activity in relation to the other states. Thus, overcoming humiliation in the mastery state will involve pleasant effort-stress (along with the unpleasant tension-stress of the humiliation until it is overcome), provided that the paratelic state is operating at the same time. If the telic state is in operation, then the effort involved will be unpleasant.

So effort stress can occur in both the telic and the paratelic (as well as other) states, although there is evidence from three independent studies (Baker, 1988; Howard, 1988; Murgatroyd, 1985) that people who are telic-dominant tend to be more problem-focussed than emotion-focussed (using these terms in the sense of Lazarus and his colleagues, e.g., Lazarus & Folkman, 1984), whereas matters are the other way around for those who are paratelic-dominant. The implication is that telic-dominant people are, on the whole, more effortful—and therefore subject to effort-stress—than paratelic-dominant people. This means that telic-dominant people are generally willing to put up with the unpleasantness of effort in order to achieve their serious goals.

One of the things that all this implies is that it is difficult to avoid stress entirely. Whether a person opts to put up with whatever form of tension-stress troubles that person at a particular time or opts to fight it in an effortful way, he or she will experience stress. The issue is whether the person would prefer to take his or her stress in the form of tension-stress or of effort-stress. There is a sense here in which the person cannot win (and, of course, if the effortful tactics the person uses to eliminate tension-stress are poorly chosen or poorly executed, then he or she may come to suffer from both types of stress simultaneously.) Fortunately, as has been shown, paratelic effort-stress is not dysphoric, and so in this sense it is possible to win after all.

Another issue is this: Do the two different types of stress lead to different types of pathology? This is a large problem, but it is already possible to discern, tentatively, the beginnings of a possible pattern, although much research is needed to see how far it can be sustained. This pattern is that tension-stress would appear to be associated more with psychopathological problems, whereas unpleasant (telic) effort-stress would appear to have more to do with medical problems. That is, tension-stress tends to have mental consequences and telic effort-stress to have somatic consequences. Thus, neurosis could be said typically to involve chronic or acute unpleasant emotions, especially anxiety, whereas the somatic consequences of stress—such as ulcers, backache (see Chapter 5 by Svebak, Mykletun and Bru), hypertension (see Chapter 7 by Spicer & Lyons) or autoimmunity—appear to emerge from situations involving prolonged effort under pressure as well as the tension that leads to this.

The relation of depression to burnout is an interesting case in point. Depression may be seen as involving some form of chronic tension that the individual has come to believe he or she can do little or nothing about and has therefore become resigned to (Apter, 1982). As a consequence, little effort is expended in an attempt to deal with the cause of the tension. In contrast, when the individual expends a great deal of energy over time but still fails to achieve what he or she seriously wanted to achieve, the result is likely to be burnout rather than depression, and burnout is associated with such somatic problems as acute fatigue. One should, of course, remind oneself that often both tension-stress and telic effort-stress are present for a prolonged period, especially when the individual is using effortful but unsuccessful strategies in the attempt to lower tension. So tension-stress will not necessarily be absent in cases of psychosomatic symptoms, and telic effort-stress will not necessarily be absent when the individual is suffering from one or another form of psychiatric syndrome.

The fact that stress can have two very different kinds of effect usually, and surprisingly, goes unremarked and unresearched. The reason is probably because two stress literatures have developed, the psychological–psychiatric on the one hand and the medical–physiological on the other, and these two literatures make rather little reference to each other. For this reason, each tends to see stress exclusively in its own terms. So the basic question of why stress sometimes has psychological consequences and sometimes has physiological consequences (and sometimes both) goes not only unanswered, but also unexamined. Yet it is one that naturally arises from the reversal theory approach.

THE METAMOTIVATIONAL LEVEL OF ANALYSIS

The fourth theme, a more fundamental one that underlies the previous three, is the key part that metamotivational states play in the psychological—and by extension, the physiological—life of the individual. Each such state constitutes a kind of internal context for behavior and a framework of meaning for construing the world. The implication is that it is essential to know which metamotivational states are operating at a given time if one is to understand the actions and functioning of the individual concerned at that time. This theme has been pursued in two different, although related, ways in reversal theory research as it relates to physical and mental health.

First of all, metamotivational state (and also state dominance) can be seen as a moderator variable that may play a crucial part in determining the outcome of various kinds of situation, manipulation, or intervention. This idea is implied in much of the work on stress as being enjoyable that is referred to above, in such work as that reported in Chapter 3 (by Lafreniere) that shows that stress is perceived in different ways in the telic and paratelic states, and in work reported in Chapter 5 (by Svebak, Mykletun, and Bru) that demonstrates that certain features of back pain are to some degree metamotivational-state–dependent. It is also an idea that has been pursued in detail at a psychophysiological level by Svebak and his colleagues in Norway, especially in relation to the telic–paratelic pair of states (see Chapter 6). A summary of all their findings, published over more than a decade, can be found in Apter and Svebak (1992). Further examples of psychobiological research involving metamotivation as a moderator variable can be found in Chapter 7 (by Spicer & Lyons), where the outcome variable is cardiovascular reactivity, and in Chapter 9 (by Cook, Gerkovich, and O'Connell), a complex study in which central nervous system activity was measured in three different ways.

Second, knowledge of metamotivational states is essential if researchers are to understand healthy and unhealthy behavior. One of the strengths of reversal theory is that it allows researchers to approach the question *Why do people perform this kind of behavior?* in a systematic and comprehensive way. That is, in attempting to answer this kind of question, researchers are led by reversal theory to consider all eight metamotivational states and the basic desires (metamotives) that they represent, together with all the different combinations of these states. In other words, it helps researchers to perform what might be referred to as metamotivational analysis.

The question of why people perform certain kinds of behavior is an important one in psychological medicine. On the one hand, as O'Connell and Brooks point out (Chapter 13), there are unhealthy behaviors, often related to addictive urges (like smoking, drug-taking, performing unsafe sexual practices), whose frequency people want to decrease. On the other hand, there are healthy behaviors (like taking exercise, eating sensibly, having regular medical check-ups) whose frequency people want to increase, at least up to some acceptable level. If the motives for both these kinds of behaviors are known, then one has some kind of handle that can be used to change behavior.

A good example of research on the metamotivational concomitants of a medically undesirable behavior is the body of work on smoking, and the attempt to quit smoking, that has been generated in Kansas City by a group of researchers based at the Midwest Research Institute and the Kansas University School of Nursing. Some of this important research is summarized in Chapter 8 of this book. Likewise, Apter and Batler, in Chapter 10, look at the metamotivational states involved in a gratuitously risky sport. On the side of more clearly desirable behavior, Apter and Spirn examine the states that lead people to donate blood (Chapter 12).

STRESS AND THE DYNAMICS OF REVERSAL

It will be realized that, from the perspective of reversal theory, the same situation can be experienced by a given individual in opposite ways; this means that, in a sense, nothing is irremediably or enduringly good or bad. Thus, as has been shown, a stimulating situation can be experienced as exciting or threatening; breaking rules can be associated with an exhilarating sense of freedom or a debilitating feeling of isolation; getting more than one gives in a friendship can lead one to experience either the pangs of guilt or the warmth of gratitude; and so on.

This brings one to the most distinctive concept of reversal theory: the pivotal idea that good and bad feelings can not only relate, in principle, to the same situation, but that such feelings can change from one to the other, suddenly and even dramatically, as reversal occurs. Furthermore, the worse the feeling before the reversal, the better it will be afterward, and vice versa (once again, the reader is referred to Figure 1).

It would not be too much to say that understanding this seeming paradox has important implications for any attempt to make sense of the dynamics of stress and health. For one thing, it shows how unhealthy behaviors may arise as attempts, frequently successful, to achieve good feelings by generating bad feelings and then converting them, through reversal, to good ones. A general strategy that has been discussed at some length elsewhere (Apter, 1992) is that of generating anxiety by provoking gratuitous risk and danger and then converting this to excitement through a reversal to the paratelic state. A common way of achieving excitement in this way is by undertaking dangerous sports, like bungee-jumping, hang-gliding, mountain-climbing, whitewater rafting, extreme skiing, and so on. The emotional switches that occur during the performance of one such sport, parachuting, are documented in Chapter 10. Of course, such sports have a healthy aspect in terms of helping to maintain physical fitness, but they can also cause injury and even death. Other ways of implementing this general anxiety-to-excitement strategy are even less healthy and even more dangerous, for example, gambling (Brown, 1991), soccer hooliganism and vandalism (Kerr, 1994), civil disobedience (McDermott, 1991), and risky sexual behavior in this age of AIDS (see Chapter 11 by Gerkovich). More on these and other dangerous behaviors can be found in Kerr, Frank-Ragan, and Brown (1993). (There is a sense too, in which humor also involves the conversion of something that might be seen as at least mildly threatening—a puzzle or dissonance—into something that is a pleasurable form of arousal; this is a point that is taken up in Chapter 14 by Svebak & Martin.)

Contrariwise, certain forms of neurosis and behavioral disorder may be seen to arise from a tendency for inappropriate reversals to occur in some domain of experience in such a way as to convert good feelings to bad in that domain. A good example would be that of sexual dysfunction in which, according to the reversal theory analysis, sexual excitement is converted to sexual anxiety when a reversal to the telic state occurs. (This might arise, e.g., when there is some perceived threat to the ability to perform adequately or when the situation comes to be seen as necessary for some purpose rather than enjoyable in itself. For a more full discussion, see Apter, 1982; Frey, 1991.) It should be noted that what reversal theory suggests here is not that anxiety inhibits sexual excitement (the common formulation), but that the anxiety is the sexual excitement perceived in the wrong mode. Another example of inappropriate reversal is that of agoraphobia, in which the mild excitement that arises from such things as being in a public place or interacting with friends becomes converted, through a reversal to the telic state, to mild anxiety (and this in turn initiates a vicious circle in which anxiety leads to anxiety about anxiety, which leads to yet further anxiety, and so on in a positive-feedback loop). An illustrative reversal theory case history of agoraphobia can be found in Murgatroyd and Apter (1986).

In general terms, reversal theory emphasizes a certain innate instability in the way in which people see situations, and therefore in the emotions that they experience in relation to them. As a consequence, it helps to understand some of the seeming inappropriateness with which people sometimes react to events. Here are a couple of examples chosen specifically because they relate to illness and health. First, one would expect that people who are ill or convalescent would feel suitably unhappy during the period concerned and that their emotions throughout would be unpleasant ones like anger and depression. Cook (1990), however, has documented, through interview and self-report, the fact that people also often admit to experiencing definitely pleasant emotions from time to time in relation to their illnesses. For instance, some people reported to Cook that their illnesses were actually fun, as this student did: "It was a fun, relaxing break from my normal routine, and I didn't have to worry about classes because it was Spring Break." Others reported on the pleasures of being cared for and cosseted (pleasant feelings in the autic and sympathy states). The second example of seeming inappropriateness concerns bereavement. One would expect, and the conventional view is, that the bereaved individual would experience nothing but grief and depression for a period after the death of a loved one. Wortman and Silver (1987), however, marshaled evidence to show that this is far from the case and that many people report periods of happiness from quite early on in the bereavement process. This would seem to be quite inexplicable unless one assumes some kind of innate experiential instability, such as that posited by reversal theory.

CONCLUSION

There are many implications of the five themes that have been introduced here, both for future research in behavioral medicine and for the practice of therapy. Perhaps the most basic of these implications is that there is a whole level of functioning, the metamotivational level, and a whole principle of change, metamotivational reversal, that play a key role in both psychological actions and psychobiological processes but that have gone largely unrecognized until the advent of reversal theory. The underlying aim of this book is to bring this level of analysis, and the various concepts developed in studying it, to the attention of those working on stress and in related fields, both pure and applied. It is also to show how research generated by this general approach can provide novel insights into a variety of entrenched problems, as well as giving rise to a whole set of new and challenging questions of its own.

REFERENCES

Apter, M. J. (1982). *The experience of motivation: The theory of psychological reversals.* London: Academic Press.

Apter, M. J. (1989). *Reversal theory: Motivation, emotion and personality.* London: Routledge.

Apter, M. J. (1991a). Reversal theory and the structure of emotional experience. In C. D. Spielberger, I. G. Sarason, Z. Kulcsar, & G. L. Van Heck (Eds.), *Stress and emotion* (Vol. 14, pp. 17–30). New York: Hemisphere.

Apter, M. J. (1991b). A structural phenomenology of stress. In C. D. Spielberger, I. G. Sarason, J. Strelau, & J. M. T. Brebner (Eds.), *Stress and anxiety* (Vol. 13, pp. 13–22). New York: Hemisphere.

Apter, M. J. (1992). *The dangerous edge: The psychology of excitement* New York: Free Press.

Apter, M. J., & Svebak, S. (1989). Stress from the reversal theory perspective. In C. D. Spielberger, I. G. Sarason, & J. Strelau (Eds.), *Stress and anxiety* (Vol. 12, pp. 39–52). New York: Hemisphere.

Apter, M. J., & Svebak, S. (1992). Reversal theory as a biological approach to individual differences. In A. Gale & M. W. Eysenck (Eds.), *Handbook of individual differences:Biological perspectives* (pp. 323–353). Chichester, England: Wiley.

Baker, J. (1988). Stress appraisals and coping with everyday hassles. In M. J. Apter, J. Kerr, & M. Cowles (Eds.), *Progress in reversal theory* (pp. 117–128). Amsterdam: North Holland.

Brown, R. I. F. (1991). Gaming, gambling and other addictive play. In J. H. Kerr & M. J. Apter (Eds.), *Adult play: A reversal theory approach* (pp. 101–118). Amsterdam: Swets & Zeitlinger.

Cook, L. (1991, June). *The experience of illness and recovery as explained by reversal theory.* Paper presented at the Fifth International Conference on Reversal Theory, Midwest Research Institute, Kansas City.

de la Pena, A. (1983). *The psychobiology of cancer: Automatization and boredom in health and disease.* New York: Praeger.

Frey, K. (1991). Sexual behavior as adult play. In J. H. Kerr & M. J. Apter (Eds.), *Adult play: A reversal theory approach* (pp. 55–69). Amsterdam: Swets & Zeitlinger.

Howard, R. (1988). Telic dominance, personality and coping. In M. J. Apter, J. Kerr, & M. Cowles (Eds.), *Progress in reversal theory* (pp. 129–142). Amsterdam: North Holland.

Kerr, J. H. (1994). *Understanding soccer hooliganism.* Buckingham, England: Open University Press.

Kerr, J. H., Frank-Ragan, E., & Brown, R. I. F. (1993). Taking risks with health. *Patient Education and Counselling, 22,* 73–80.

Lafreniere, K. D. (1993). Arousability and telic dominance. In J. H. Kerr, S. Murgatroyd, & M. J. Apter (Eds.), *Advances in reversal theory* (pp. 257–266). Amsterdam: Swets & Zeitlinger.

Lazarus, R. S., & Folkman, S. (1984). *Stress, appraisal, and coping.* New York: Springer.

Martin, R. A., Kuiper, N. A., & Olinger, L. (1988). Telic versus paratelic dominance as a moderator of stress. In M. J. Apter, J. Kerr, & M. Cowles (Eds.), *Progress in reversal theory* (pp. 91–106). Amsterdam: North Holland.

Martin, R. A., Kuiper, N. A., Olinger, L. J., & Dobbin, J. (1987). Is stress always bad? Telic versus paratelic dominance as a stress moderating variable. *Journal of Personality and Social Psychology, 53,* 970–982.

McDermott, M. R. (1991). Negativism as play: Proactive rebellion in young adult life. In J. H. Kerr & M. J. Apter (Eds.), *Adult play: A reversal theory approach* (pp. 87–99). Amsterdam: Swets & Zeitlinger.

Murgatroyd, S. (1985). The nature of telic dominance. In M. J. Apter, D. Fontana, & S. Murgatroyd (Eds.), *Reversal theory: Applications and developments* (pp. 20–41). Cardiff, Wales: University College Cardiff Press.

Murgatroyd, S., & Apter, M. J. (1986). A structural-phenomenological approach to eclectic psychotherapy. In J. C. Norcross (Ed.), *Handbook of eclectic psychotherapy* (pp. 260–281). New York: Brunner/Mazel.

Svebak, S. (1991a). One state's agony, the other's delight: Perspectives on coping and musculoskeletal complaints. In C. D. Spielberger, I. G. Sarason, J. Strelau, & J. M. T. Brebner (Eds.), *Stress and anxiety* (Vol. 13, pp. 215–229). New York: Hemisphere.

Svebak, S. (1991b). The role of effort in stress and emotion. In C. D. Spielberger, I. G. Sarason, Z. Kulcsar, & G. L. Van Heck (Eds.), *Stress and emotion* (Vol. 14, pp. 121–134). New York: Hemisphere.

Svebak, S. (1993). The development of the Tension and Effort Stress Inventory (TESI). In J. H. Kerr, S. Murgatroyd, & M. J. Apter (Eds.), *Advances in reversal theory* (pp. 189–204). Amsterdam: Swets & Zeitlinger.

Wortman, C. B., & Silver, R. C. (1987). Coping with irrevocable loss. In G. R. VandenBos & B. K. Bryant (Eds.), *Cataclysms, crises, and catastrophes: Psychology in action* (Master Lecture Series, Vol. 6, pp. 189–235). Washington, DC: American Psychological Association.

II

THE EFFECTS OF STRESS

3

Paratelic Dominance
and the Appraisal of Stressful Events

Kathryn D. Lafreniere

Transactional models of stress emphasize the idea that it is the perception of events as stressful rather than the characteristics of the objective events that determines whether negative mental and physical health consequences will ensue. This investigation was designed to examine the relationship between objectively experienced daily hassles and subjective appraisals of these events as stressful, within a reversal theory framework. Undergraduate student volunteers completed questionnaire measures of daily hassles, perceived stress, paratelic dominance, and somatic state. It was hypothesized that paratelic-dominant and telic-dominant individuals would not differ in the number of daily hassles reported. Telic-dominant participants were expected to appraise the events as being more stressful, however, and thereby to experience more deleterious effects of the stressors. Results indicated that paratelic-dominant and telic-dominant people did not differ significantly in their self-reports of daily hassles. Telic-dominant individuals reported greater perceived stress when experiencing a high number of daily hassles as compared with those who were paratelic-dominant. Thus, paratelic dominance appears to exert a stress-buffering effect under conditions of high daily hassles. Additional findings based on Paratelic Dominance × Gender interactions and relationships between dominance and mode are also discussed.

THE APPRAISAL OF STRESSFUL EVENTS

Background and Rationale

This investigation is based on the transactional model of stress developed by Richard Lazarus and his colleagues (Lazarus & Folkman, 1984; Lazarus & Launier, 1978). Central to their model is the idea of appraisal of stressful events. When confronted with a potentially stressful event, an individual is thought to make a primary appraisal, evaluating the stressor as irrelevant, benign–positive, or stressful. An event that involves harm, loss, threat, or challenge will be appraised as stressful, according to this approach. When a stressful appraisal is made, the individual then goes on to make a secondary appraisal, in which she or he evaluates what can be done to cope with the stressor (Lazarus & Folkman, 1984).

Martin and his colleagues at the University of Western Ontario (Martin, Kuiper, Olinger, & Dobbin, 1987) examined telic dominance as a stress-moderating variable and showed that telic-dominant individuals seem to be adversely affected by even low levels of stress but that paratelic-dominant people do well under higher levels of stress. Their results led these authors to speculate that telic-dominant people might evaluate arousing situations as threats and paratelic-dominant individuals might see the same situations as challenges (Martin et al., 1987).

In a previous investigation, Lafreniere (1991) attempted to examine possible stress-moderating effects of telic–paratelic dominance and did not observe the stress-moderating effects that Martin et al. (1987) reported. One possible reason why the effects shown by Martin et al. were not reproduced was that this study measured daily hassles–type stress in university students shortly before they were due to write their mid-term examinations, which is undoubtedly a time of heavy exposure to student-related hassles. This might have been reflected in a lack of variability in response, which might, in turn, have contributed to the inability to detect the hypothesized interactions with telic dominance in predicting adverse consequences of stress.

A further problem with the Lafreniere (1991) study likely arose from restricting measurement of telic–paratelic dominance to total scores on the Telic Dominance Scale (TDS; Murgatroyd, Rushton, Apter, & Ray, 1978). Other potentially relevant indicators of telic dominance (e.g., the Serious-Mindedness subscale of the TDS) did not show adequate internal consistency reliability in Lafreniere's sample and thus could not be used.

This investigation was designed to overcome these methodological shortcomings by testing student participants during a less stressful point in the academic year and by using new and reliable measures of telic dominance and telic–paratelic state. The main objective of the study was to determine whether telic-dominant individuals would report experiencing more stress as a function of increased exposure to daily hassles in comparison with paratelic-dominant individuals. Specifically, it was expected that telic-dominant and paratelic-dominant people would report similar levels of daily hassles but that telic-dominant individuals would be more likely to perceive these events as stressful (i.e., as threats), whereas paratelic-dominant individuals would perceive them as challenges. In addition, the relationship between telic–paratelic dominance and operative metamotivational mode (i.e., as participants began the study) was examined.

METHOD

One hundred forty-one undergraduate student volunteers, both men and women, were recruited from Introductory Psychology classes at a medium-sized Canadian university. The study was conducted early in the fall semester, well before examination periods, and therefore baseline levels of student-related stress were not expected to be unduly high. Participants completed a questionnaire package consisting of the following measures:

1 *The Paratelic Dominance Scale* (PDS; Cook & Gerkovich, 1993). The PDS is a 30-item measure of telic–paratelic dominance that yields three subscale scores (Playfulness, Spontaneity, and Arousal Seeking) as well as a total paratelic dominance score. The internal reliability of PDS subscales was established in initial standardization samples, in which alpha coefficients ranging from .75 to .87 were reported (Cook & Gerkovich, 1993).

2 *The Somatic State Questionnaire* (SSQ; Cook, Gerkovich, Potocky, O'Connell, & Hoffman, 1991). The SSQ is a 12-item self-report measure of telic–paratelic state that has been demonstrated to show acceptable internal reliability and validity (Cook, Gerkovich, Potocky, & O'Connell, 1993). In this study, it was used to measure the metamotivational mode that was operative as respondents began their participation. It appeared first in the questionnaire package so that it would not be influenced by the participants' responses to measures of hassles and perceived stress (presuming that most students worked through the inventories in the order in which they were presented).

3 *The Inventory of College Students' Recent Life Experiences* (ICSRLE; Kohn, Lafreniere, & Gurevich, 1990). This is a measure of daily-hassles stress that was specifically designed for use with college or university students. An important feature of this inventory is that it does not contain items that reflect the distressed physical and mental responses to stress that the inventory is intended to predict (e.g., items pertaining to physical illness and substance use do not appear). Thus, it can be used to determine the physical and mental health consequences of exposure to everyday stressors without artificially inflating the relationship between stress and distressed response. It was designed in such a way that respondents can report everyday events that have occurred to them without necessarily defining these events as stressors or hassles. Thus, it is well-suited for use in this investigation, which attempted to separate exposure to potentially stressful events from distressed response to those events.

4 *The Perceived Stress Scale* (Cohen, Kamarack, & Mermelstein, 1983). This is a measure of appraised stress that includes items such as "In the last month, how often have you felt nervous and 'stressed'?" and "In the last month, how often have you been able to control irritations in your life?" It was positioned at the end of the questionnaire so that items asking respondents to appraise their level of stress would not influence their reactions to the hassles-exposure measure (again, presuming that they worked through the questionnaire in order).

INVESTIGATION RESULTS AND WHAT IS INFERRED

The PDS and its subscales showed fairly high internal reliability in this study, with Cronbach's alpha coefficients ranging from .79 for Playfulness to .87 for total PDS. Means and alphas obtained for the PDS and its subscales were consistent with those reported by Cook and Gerkovich (1993) in previous standardization samples. The SSQ was also adequately reliable, with alpha coefficients ranging from .63 to .65. The ICSRLE hassles measure and its subscales were generally reliable in this investigation, with the exception of one subscale, Assorted Annoyances ($\alpha = .39$). This subscale consists of miscellaneous student-related hassles, and its low reliability is therefore unsurprising. It was not included in any subsequent data analyses. All other ICSRLE subscales showed adequate internal consistency, with alphas ranging from .72 to .86. The Perceived Stress Scale also showed fairly high internal consistency, with an alpha reliability coefficient of .85.

High versus low scorers on the PDS, based on a median split, were identified as representing paratelic-dominant and telic-dominant individuals. High and low PDS scorers were compared on the hassles measure, its subscales, and perceived stress. Individuals identified as being paratelic-dominant did not differ significantly from those who were telic-dominant in their reporting of daily hassles. This was true for the total hassles score, as well as for each of the hassles subscales. An examination of each of the PDS subscales revealed only two instances of paratelic–telic differences in hassles reporting. Individuals who scored in the *serious* direction of the Playful subscale reported significantly more social mistreatment hassles than did more playful people, $t(138) = 2.17$, $p < .05$. High scorers on PDS Arousal Seeking reported more friendship problems than did those who were low in Arousal Seeking, $t(139) = 2.32$, $p < .05$. Overall, though, telic-dominant and paratelic-dominant individuals seemed to experience similar amounts of hassles-based stress.

The interactive effects of paratelic dominance and hassles exposure on perceived stress were examined to test for paratelic–telic differences in the appraisal of stress. In addition to a large main effect for low versus high hassles reporting, $F(1, 98) = 37.85$, $p < .001$, there was a significant interaction between level of hassles and paratelic dominance, $F(1, 98) = 3.95$, $p < .05$. As shown in Figure 1A, under low exposure to hassles, paratelic-dominant participants were somewhat higher in perceived stress than telic-dominant participants, whereas under high hassles-exposure, the opposite effect was seen. Here, telic-dominant individuals were more distressed by the effects of hassles-based stress. This result supported the principal hypothesis and is consistent with the speculation by Martin et al. (1987) that paratelic-dominant individuals may be more likely to perceive events as challenges and telic-dominant people appraise the same events as threats and are thus more negatively affected by them.

An examination of the same relationship, using only the Playfulness subscale of the PDS, revealed a similar interactive effect, $F(1, 97) = 6.38$, $p < .05$. Under

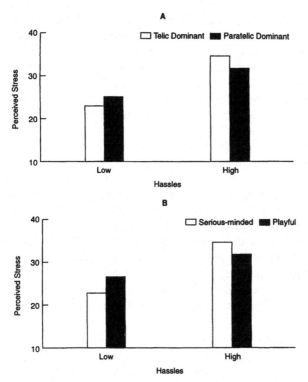

Figure 1 Perceived stress as a function of daily hassles, paratelic dominance, and playfulness.

low exposure to hassles, individuals who scored high in playfulness showed greater perceived stress than those who were identified as more serious. Under high levels of hassles, the opposite effect occurred, as depicted in Figure 1B. Thus, the effect seems to be fairly robust and related to the playfulness component of paratelic dominance. No significant interactive effects were obtained for the spontaneous and arousal-seeking dimensions of paratelic dominance.

Other theoretically consistent findings emerged when the metamotivational modes of participants at the time of participation were examined in relation to the hassles and stress measures. Individuals in the negativistic mode were more likely than people in the conformist mode to report higher levels of hassles overall, $t(139) = -2.87$, $p < .005$, as well as more hassles related to social mistreatment, $t(139) = -2.07$, $p < .05$; romantic problems, $t(139) = -3.10$, $p < .005$; and friendship problems, $t(139) = -3.08$, $p < .005$.

The negativistic versus conformist differences in hassles reporting might have reflected differences in subjective appraisal. Although the ICSRLE hassles measure attempts to minimize the influence of appraisal, it is really impossible to do away with it altogether. Thus, a person who is in a particularly angry and defiant state might be more likely to endorse hassles such as "being taken

advantage of," "having your contributions overlooked," and "conflicts with pro-
fessors" than would those in a conformist state, quite independently of the
objective reality of those events. A second possibility is that heavy exposure to
hassles elicits more frequent engagement of the negativistic mode, thus making
it more likely that highly hassled individuals will be captured in the negativistic
mode during the course of an investigation. Although the possibility also exists
that the act of completing measures of hassles and perceived stress might elicit
a reversal to the negativistic mode, this potential confound was minimized in
this study by having participants fill out the SSQ first (thereby capturing their
current metamotivational mode).

An unexpected finding was that of a significant interactive relationship between paratelic dominance and gender in predicting romantic problems hassles,
$F(1, 102) = 11.86, p < .001$. As illustrated in Figure 2A, men who were paratelic-
dominant reported more romantic problems than did men who were telic-
dominant. For women, the opposite effect occurred, with telic-dominant women
scoring higher on romantic problems hassles than did paratelic-dominant women.
A similar interaction emerged for the Playfulness subscale of the PDS, where
serious-minded women and playful men again fared worse than their counterparts
in terms of romantic difficulties, $F(1, 101) = 5.74, p < .05$ (see Figure 2A).

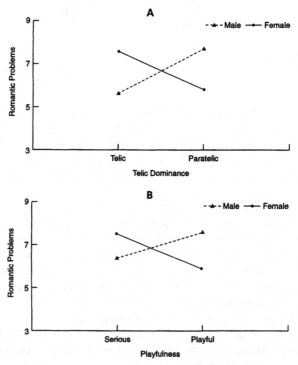

Figure 2 Romantic problems as a function of paratelic dominance, playfulness, and
gender.

One possible interpretation of these results is that traditional gender role socialization might lead women to take a more committed and serious approach to romantic relationships, whereas men would be seen (at least stereotypically) to prefer a more casual and uncommitted approach. Thus, serious-minded men who plan for the future and are arousal avoiders (i.e., telic-dominant) would meet the expectations of many women and thus would be less likely to experience as many romantic difficulties in comparison with men who take a more casual approach. In a sense, these results suggest that individuals who operate outside of stereotypical gender roles with regard to relationships (women who are playful and men who are serious) fare better romantically than those who adopt a more traditional approach.

There are, of course, a number of limitations to this interpretation. For one thing, it presupposes a completely heterosexual sample. Because relationship issues were not the focus of this study, background information regarding sexual orientation was not collected. Although heterosexual students undoubtedly comprised the majority of the sample, it is virtually certain that some participants were responding on the basis of their relationships with their homosexual partners.

Another difficulty with this line of speculation is that it relates to a dyadic issue but is based on observation of only one half of the dyad. Thus, an interesting question would be whether the serious-minded women in the study actually had difficulties that stemmed from being involved with men whom they perceived as being too casual and whether the playful men who reported more romantic problems tended to be paired with serious women. The results of this investigation suggest that further study of the implications of telic–paratelic dominance for romantic relationships, as well as interpersonal relationships in general, seems to be warranted.

In conducting this investigation, another focus of interest was on the relationship between telic dominance and the actual metamotivational mode of the respondents during initial participation in the study. Although one would anticipate a significant positive relationship between dominance and mode, it is interesting to observe the proportion of participants who were in a state that was opposite to their dominant one. An examination of the top, middle, and bottom third of scorers on the PDS and SSQ yields the results that are depicted in Figure 3.

Although there was a highly significant association between paratelic dominance and mode, $\chi^2(4, N = 141) = 31.65$, $p < .0001$, a full 22% of highly telic-dominant participants were in a highly paratelic mode when approaching the study. Ten percent of the highly paratelic-dominant group began the task in a highly telic mode. This finding supports the reversal theory conceptualization of dominance as reflecting an individual's propensity to spend relatively more time in a particular mode, yet at the same time being fully capable of switching to the mode completely opposite to their dominant mode.

Interestingly, where such opposite effects occurred, they did so in this di-

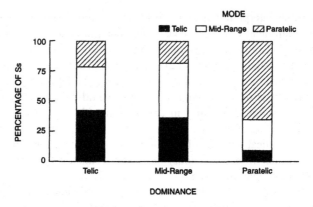

Figure 3   Relationship between dominance and metamotivational mode while participating.

rection: A greater proportion of telic-dominant people operated in the paratelic mode while beginning this task as compared with the proportion of paratelic-dominant individuals who operated within the telic mode. This is surprising, in that it is generally assumed that participation in a research investigation will be perceived as a fairly serious task for most individuals. Although the respondents did appear to take the task seriously (i.e., they completed the entire questionnaire and were observed to work alone and diligently), participation in this study might have brought about a switch to the paratelic mode for some individuals. For many students expecting their usual Introductory Psychology lecture, participation in an investigation that was introduced as being entirely voluntary and unrelated to the course or their evaluation in it might have been experienced by them as a kind of game (i.e., in the paratelic mode). This leads one to speculate that many research investigations that require students to fill out self-report inventories during class time might be experienced in a similar fashion and that metamotivational mode might influence responding to measures of mood, attitude, and other psychological constructs.

CONCLUSION

In summary, then, the results of this investigation were in line with those reported by Martin et al. (1987) and seem to support the proposition that similar events might be regarded as threats by telic-dominant individuals and as challenges by those who are paratelic-dominant. As a result, paratelic dominance appears to buffer some of the effects of being exposed to a high level of everyday stressors.

Some findings from this investigation support the construct validity of the Negativistic subscale of the SSQ by showing that while in the negativistic state individuals report more hassles in general, as well as in specific problem areas that relate to the negativism construct.

The finding that playful men and serious women reported greater problems with romance was both interesting and unexpected, and might be worth a more detailed consideration in future research that examines telic–paratelic dominance in relation to interpersonal relationships.

Finally, the observation that telic and paratelic dominance were highly associated with mode (i.e., temporary state), but that some individuals who scored in the extremely high range on the dominance measure were also found to score extremely highly on the opposite mode, lends support to the reversal theory conceptualization of dominance, as distinct from trait (Apter, 1989; Apter & Apter-Desselles, 1993). Because paratelic dominance was shown to exert a stress-buffering effect, facilitating reversals to the paratelic mode might be an effective intervention in the process of making stressful appraisals, for both paratelic- and telic-dominant people.

REFERENCES

Apter, M. J. (1989). *Reversal theory: Motivation, emotion, and personality*. London: Routledge.

Apter, M. J., & Apter-Desselles, M. L. (1993) The personality of the patient: Going beyond the trait concept. *Patient Education and Counselling, 22*, 107–114.

Cohen, S., Kamarack, T., & Mermelstein, R. (1983). A global measure of perceived stress. *Journal of Health and Social Behavior, 24*, 385–396.

Cook, M. R., & Gerkovich, M. M. (1993). The development of a Paratelic Dominance Scale. In J. H. Kerr, S. Murgatroyd, & M. J. Apter (Eds.), *Advances in reversal theory* (pp. 177–188). Amsterdam: Swets & Zeitlinger.

Cook, M. R., Gerkovich, M. M., Potocky, M., & O'Connell, K. A. (1993). Instruments for the assessment of reversal theory states. *Patient Education and Counseling, 22*, 99–106.

Cook, M. R., Gerkovich, M. M., Potocky, M., O'Connell, K. A., & Hoffman, S. J. (1991, June). *Progress toward the development of instruments to measure reversal theory constructs*. Paper presented at the 5th International Conference on Reversal Theory and Health, Kansas City, MO.

Kohn, P. M., Lafreniere, K. D., & Gurevich, M. (1990). The Inventory of College Students' Recent Life Experiences: A decontaminated hassles scale for a special population. *Journal of Behavioral Medicine, 13*, 619–630.

Lafreniere, K. D. (1991, June). *The stress-moderating effects of telic dominance and arousability*. Paper presented at the 5th International Conference on Reversal Theory and Health, Kansas City, MO.

Lazarus, R. S., & Folkman, S. (1984). *Stress, appraisal, and coping*. New York: Springer.

Lazarus, R. S., & Launier, R. (1978). Stress-related transactions between person and environment. In L. A. Pervin & M. Lewis (Eds.), *Perspectives in interactional psychology* (pp. 287–327). New York: Plenum.

Martin, R. A., Kuiper, N. A., Olinger, L. J., & Dobbin, J. (1987). Is stress always bad? Telic versus paratelic dominance as a stress-moderating variable. *Journal of Personality and Social Psychology, 53*, 970–982.

Murgatroyd, S., Rushton, C., Apter, M. J., & Ray, R. E. (1978). The development of the Telic Dominance Scale. *Journal of Personality Assessment, 42*, 519–528.

4

Tension- and Effort-Stress as Predictors of Academic Performance

Sven Svebak

Students who prepared for the introductory psychology examination at the University of Bergen were recruited to a prospective study of predictors of academic performance on the exam. Two samples of students were studied in separate Spring terms. Measures were obtained to test the hypothesis that stressors provoke tension-stress and that increasing efforts helps to reduce tension-stress. A second hypothesis related to the prospective nature of the two studies and predicted better performance among students who invested much effort and experienced low tension-stress.

Results from both studies yielded high coefficients of correlation between scores on strength of stressors and of intensity of efforts to cope. Moreover, in Study 1, relatively low effort despite high stress was found among students who reported high tension-stress and who predicted poor performance on the exam. The significance of type of strategy and not only of amount of effort-stress was indicated in Study 1 by a prevalence of problem-focused coping among successful students. These students scored particularly low on sullenness and guilt 4 weeks ahead of the exam in Study 1. They were also characterized by the absence of excitement as well as by the presence of anxiety 1 week ahead of the exam in Study 2. Overall, these studies confirmed that stressors tend to induce tension-stress and that effort-stress is inversely related to tension-stress. Also, quality of performance was good with high effort-stress. Four weeks ahead of the exam, tension-stress was inversely related to the quality of the subsequent performance, whereas tension-stress in the form of anxiety (telic goal-directedness) was a promising sign just before the exam. At this point in time, excitement (high arousal when in the paratelic state of playfulness) predicted poor performance.

The concept of tension-stress may be defined as a discrepancy between the preferred and actual level of a variable operated on by a metamotivational state.

The immediate experience of tension-stress takes the form of unpleasant emotion from among the range of basic emotions defined in reversal theory and presented in the introductory chapter (Chapter 1) by Frey. Moreover, any normal attempt to reduce tension requires some kind of effortful activity that, therefore, constitutes a secondary form of stress that has been labeled effort-stress. (A detailed account of the relations between effort-stress and tension-stress is given in Chapter 2.)

The purpose of this chapter is to review findings from two studies in which university students invested varying degrees of effort to cope with the process of preparing for an impending and important exam. Two hypotheses were tested. Hypothesis 1 assumed that stressors provoke tension-stress and that increasing efforts helps to reduce tension-stress. Hypothesis 2 predicted a positive correlation between degree of effort in preparing for the exam and the quality of the subsequent performance. This is to say that when the individual is faced with a major challenge, demand, or threat, two beneficial outcomes are expected from the reversal theory position: One is that effortful striving tends to be invested to reduce tension-stress, and the other is, of course, the increased probability of successful coping with the external stressor. However, the eventual outcome when coping with an impending exam is the evaluation of one's performance after the exam is completed. The prospective structure of the studies reported here meant that the predictive value of tension-stress and efforts to prepare over the weeks before the exam was tested with regard to subsequent quality of performance.

The concept of effort-stress has been phenomenologically defined within reversal theory as the experience of expenditure of effort in order to reduce tension-stress. This is to say that effort is expended to overcome some cause of unpleasant emotion. Traditionally, the concept of effort has been introduced by use of a large number of energetically oriented terms in psychology. These terms have partly oriented to the central nervous system (arousal), information processing (attention, capacity), or the autonomic nervous system (activation). Terms such as *effort, vigilance,* and *fatigue* have a more integrative orientation by making reference to the central, autonomic, and peripheral nervous systems. Despite the diverse orientation to the concept of effort adopted by work physiologists, industrial engineers, and psychologists, they all agree that physical demands are involved and that energy is expended in effort-demanding processes. Whereas the professional work physiologists may regard effort as the amount of energy expended on a time-locked task, ergonomic and industrial engineers define effort in terms of work output per time unit, and psychologists in applied settings often regard effort as a synonym for perceived task difficulty (see Hockey, Gaillard & Coles, 1986, and Svebak, 1991, for more extensive discussions of nonphenomenological orientations to the concept of effort).

Different assumptions about the relation between emotions and the expenditure of effort have been published over the past 40 years, and in some ways derive from the older distinction by Cannon (1927) between crisis situation and crisis response. Activation theorists incorporated this theme within the more general concept of activation, implying that the expenditure of effort is one way of boosting physiological activation. The idea of optimal arousal was one of several cornerstones in their reasoning. Moderate levels of effort were assumed to give rise to pleasant emotions, whereas too high or too low levels of effortful striving (supposedly involving very high or very low levels of activation, respectively) would give rise to unpleasant emotions (e.g., Duffy, 1957; Hebb, 1955; see also Cannon, 1927). The inverted-U–shaped relationship with activation was extended into the fields of performance quality as well as focus of attention (the so-called cue function; Hebb, 1955). All these assumptions are illustrated in Figure 1A.

A somewhat different formulation of the relation between metabolic activity and hedonic tone was introduced by Obrist (1981), who investigated these phenomena within a cardiovascular research context that manipulated task difficulty. His concept of effortful active coping implied that active coping elicits cardiac activation (heart rate and systolic blood pressure) in excess of metabolic

A

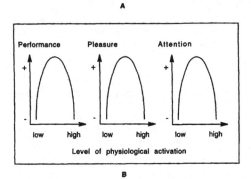

B

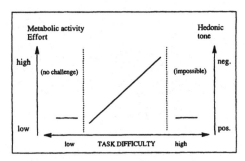

Figure 1 Illustrations of assumptions about inverted-U–shaped relations between level of physiological activation and quality of task performance as well as hedonic tone and attention, showing that medium levels of activation relate to maximal performance, pleasant emotions, and good focus of attention, respectively (A). An alternative position is presented (B) where metabolic activity, effort, and intensity of unpleasant emotions are all expected to show linear relations with increasing levels of task difficulty, and these linear relations are expected to collapse when tasks are perceived to be within ranges that are very easy or impossibly difficult.

demands. This psychobiological discrepancy was termed *additional heart rate* by Strømme, Wikeby, Blix, and Ursin (1978) and was attributed to the psychological activation of the heart muscle because of increase of mental effort. Obrist argued that the relation between effort and metabolic activity is a linear function that disappears when tasks are either very easy or extremely difficult. Ursin and Murison (1983), however, argued that strong activation has definite unpleasant aspects to it. These views may be seen as somewhat different from the inverted-U curve and are incorporated into Figure 1B where they are all related to task difficulty.

Although one may argue that there is a degree of similarity between the assumptions illustrated in Figures 1A and 1B, there is a remarkable contrast between these assumptions and the proposed relationship between hedonic tone and degree of effort (relative to the power of the actual stressor) given in Figure 2. According to reversal theory, a central phenomenological characteristic of stressors is their ability to induce unpleasant emotions (tension-stress), and the expenditure of effort (effort-stress) aims at overcoming this tension. In Figure 2, the analogy of the piston within a cylinder illustrates the relative balance of the opposing forces due to the stressor and the counteracting effort-stress. The net outcome of these opposing forces defines whether there will be "space" for tension-stress or not. With high stressor-force, relative to the counteracting effort-stress, the position of the piston in Figure 2 moves to the right, creating much space for tension-stress. With high opposing power of effort-stress, relative to the power of the stressor, the position of the piston shifts to the left and leaves reduced space for tension-stress.

The choice of strategy is a complicating factor in this dynamic relationship because much effort can be invested in a poor strategy. One example would be

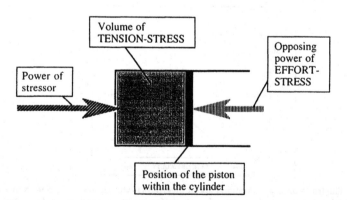

Figure 2 Illustration of the assumptions in reversal theory of the dynamic phenomenological relationships between power of stressors, tension-stress (unpleasant emotions), and the opposing power of effort-stress invested to counteract the power of a stressor. Note that in this analogy of a cylinder, the position of the piston can shift toward the right or toward the left, depending on the relative balance of the two opposing powers and thus provides a larger or smaller space, respectively, representing tension-stress.

the student who is fearful when faced with the stress of an impending exam. From a rational point of view, preparation to cope successfully with the exam involves such activities as reading the relevant textbooks and attending relevant lectures, whereas the student may instead spend much time and energy talking to friends about fear of failure. This expenditure of effort, although maladaptive, may nevertheless help to reduce tension-stress and provide an illusion of transitory coping (note the distinction between problem-focused vs. emotion-focused ways of coping, proposed by Lazarus & Folkman, 1984). A related way of short-term coping with tension-stress is the low-effort strategy of drug-taking that pharmacologically takes away tension-stress for as long as the effect of the drug. However, it fails to increase the ability to actually cope with the task of preparing for the exam and, thus, again represents a form of self-deception.

The two studies reviewed in this chapter tested the hypotheses that (a) the expenditure of effort to prepare for a forthcoming exam helps in reducing if not completely overcoming tension-stress (illustrated in the shift of the position of the piston toward the left in the cylinder of Figure 2) and (b) that the performance on the exam also improves with increasing effort-stress. This latter hypothesis involves the premise that effort is invested intelligently on the development of knowledge and skills that are actually tested on the exam. Both studies were reported to the University of Bergen as part of a larger 2-year project that aimed at evaluating and improving the quality of the learning environment throughout all faculties at this university (Svebak, 1988).

STUDY 1

Method

Participants   The study recruited 102 students who had signed up for the examination in Introductory Psychology. The normal time to prepare for this exam in Norway is 1.5 years, and approximately 25–30% of the students are rewarded with marks that permit them to enter the 5-year professional training program that qualifies them to become licensed psychologists in Norway. This means that for most of the students this exam is highly ego-involving and very competitive. Most of the subjects were female ($N = 84$), and the overall mean age was 23.6 years.

Surveys and Design   All participants were given a set of questionnaires 4 weeks ahead of the exam, and the deadline for return of the forms was 2 weeks before the exam. Participants were identified by name on the questionnaires, which meant that performance on the exam could be related to their responses to these survey measures in a prospective way, blind to their subsequent performance on the exam.

One part of the survey consisted of a short version of the Tension and Effort Stress Inventory (TESI) asking for estimates on magnitude of stressor because of the impending exam and amount of effort invested to cope. Eight items also assessed the basic forms of unpleasant emotions as defined in reversal theory (see Chapter 5 and Svebak, 1993).

Differences among the students in so-called ways of coping were assessed by use of the 66-item student version of this scale (Folkman & Lazarus, 1985). Subscales provide separate scores for problem-focused coping, wishful thinking, distancing, seeking social support, focusing on the positive sides, self-blame, tension reduction, and avoidance of problem disclosure to others. Differences in scores on these subscales were taken as indicators of effort in relation to different types of strategy.

Another scale included in the survey is known as Need for Cognition (Cacioppo & Petty, 1982). It was assumed that individual differences in the willingness to invest effort in preparing for academic excellence would be reflected in responses to this scale. The 18 items relate to the intrinsic need for spending time and effort on challenging tasks.

A fourth scale also related to strategy and is known as the Barratt Impulsiveness Scale (BIS-10; Barratt, 1965). This scale has 34 items and provides three different measures of impulsiveness (cognitive, nonplanning, motor). It was assumed that impulsiveness of all three kinds would present different types of interference with task demands over the course of preparing for the exam. Low scores on impulsiveness were assumed to facilitate investment of effort according to a goal-directed plan.

Students were grouped according to the independent outcome measure of academic achievement on the exam (overall mark for 2 exam days). Five groups were formed to reflect the fact that some of the students failed to show up for the exam (absent, $n = 12$), some took part but failed to pass (failed, $n = 27$), some passed with a range of poor marks (3.1–3.5; bad, $n = 17$), some students were moderately successful but failed to obtain grades that permitted enrollment in the professional psychology program (3.0–2.6; medium, $n = 22$), and the rest of the students performed very well (2.5 or better; good, $n = 24$).

Data analyses were performed on the mainframe university computer using SPSS software for Pearson's product–moment coefficients of correlation, one-way analyses of variance (ANOVAs), and discriminant analyses.

Results

The tendency for a stressor to provoke counteracting effort-stress was clearly supported in this participant sample where these two measures yielded a highly significant coefficient of correlation ($r = .57$, $p < .001$). The magnitude of the current stressor tended to be high among students who reported anxiety ($r = .27$, $p < .035$), anger ($r = .28$, $p < .025$), and sullenness ($r = .40$, $p < .001$). Tension-stress is assumed to reflect a discrepancy between amount of perceived stress and the degree of counteracting efforts invested to cope. The score on discrepancy between stress and effort (tension score) correlated significantly with boredom (r = .32, p <.01), humiliation (r = .24, p < .05), and guilt (r = .27, p < .04).

Of particular interest was the prospective ability of the survey to predict performance on the exam. Results from one-way ANOVAs confirmed that there were only marginally different perceptions among the five groups of the magnitude of the stressor (the forthcoming exam) in the 2- to 4-week period ahead of the exam, $F(4, 95)$ = 2.22, p < .072. Figure 3 shows that the students on the average rated the stressor to be in the range of 5 to 6 on a 7-point scale (0 = *no stress*, 7 = *very high stress*). A more clearly significant group difference was found for amount of effort invested in coping with the impending stressor, $F(4, 95)$ = 3.22, p < .016. Relatively little effort was reported by those students who later decided not to show up at the exam. Tension scores (discrepancy between stressor and effort scores) were also significant predictors of the subsequent academic achievements. The discrepancy was particularly high among those who ended up being absent for the exam, whereas particularly low discrepancy scores were found for the group of most successful students, $F(4, 95)$ = 3.34, p < .013.

Scores on ways of coping showed that only self-blame was a significant predictor of subsequent academic achievement, $F(4, 95)$ = 3.32, p < 0.14, owing to relatively low scores among the most successful students and high scores among those who failed to show up at the exam. A corresponding group difference emerged for scores on the BIS-10 subscale on cognitive impulsivity, $F(4, 97)$ = 3.05, p < .021, and those who were most successful scored low on the average on cognitive impulsivity, whereas those who failed to show up for the

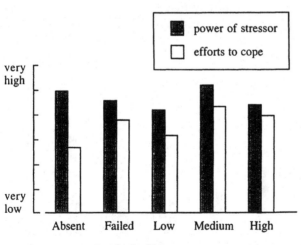

Figure 3 Illustration of mean scores for estimates of the strength of the impending stressor (forthcoming exam) and the amount of efforts invested to cope with this stressor among students grouped according to subsequent academic achievement (see text for details).

exam scored high. Similarly, those who were most successful in academic achievement scored relatively high on the Need for Cognition scale, $F(4, 95) = 2.47$, $p < .05$.

Whereas information on the discrepancy between magnitude of stressor and of efforts invested to cope provides no information on the quality of tension-stress, the results that are illustrated in Figure 4 provide such qualitative information. There was a relatively stable trend for high scores on all eight items on negative emotions among those who later decided not to show up at the exam, whereas the most successful students tended to score relatively low on all types of unpleasant emotions. However, only scores for sullenness, $F(4, 95) = 3.08$, $p < .020$, and guilt, $F(4, 95) = 2.52$, $p < .046$, yielded significant group differences.

Finally, discriminant analyses for predictors of performance in Study 1 confirmed that relatively successful students scored low on self-blame and guilt but high on need for cognition, whereas the opposite trends were seen for the less successful students (81% of students were correctly classified according to this function).

STUDY 2

Method

Participants and Design The study was replicated 1 year later with some modifications. The study population again consisted of students who signed up for the Introductory Psychology examination. At this time 83 students completed the forms that, on this occasion, were returned only 1 week ahead of the

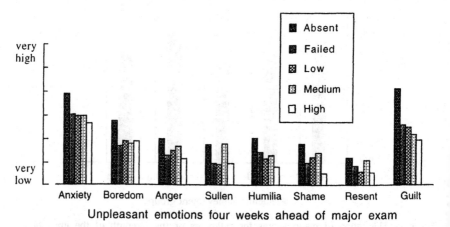

Figure 4 Illustration of mean scores for eight basic unpleasant emotions 2 to 4 weeks ahead of an important exam, with students grouped according to subsequent academic achievement (see text for details).

exam. Because the exam was so close, the survey was kept shorter: The Ways of Coping and Need for Cognition scales and BIS-10 were all excluded (around 130 items) and, instead, the complete version of the TESI was used (see Chapter 5 and Svebak, 1993). This version includes separate items for stressors due to work, family, finance, and one's own body, and a corresponding set of items asks for estimates on the degree of effort invested to cope. Eight items on pleasant emotions were also included according to the range of basic pleasant emotions in human experience, as defined in reversal theory (see Chapter 1 by Frey). Two time frames were given for students' estimates. The first asked students to make judgments in terms of the past 7 days, then a corresponding version of the inventory asked for average estimates on stressors, efforts to cope, and emotions over the past 12 months.

Groups were formed retrospectively on the basis of performance on the exam, including also a group of students who did not show up for the exam. As in Study 1, five groups were formed (absent, $n = 24$; failed, $n = 21$; low, $n = 11$; medium, $n = 18$; high, $n = 9$). Statistical analyses followed the principles applied in the data analyses of Study 1.

Results

Highly significant positive coefficients of correlation were found for the association of stressor scores with effort-stress ($r = .72$, $p < .0004$, for overall mean scores on stressors with efforts to cope; see Table 1 for details). This meant that, by and large, there was a marked tendency for a stressor to elicit efforts to cope with it. This trend appeared to be stressor-specific; for example, scores on stressors due to family were not related to efforts to cope with the academic stressor (see Table 1).

Results from ANOVAs confirmed that work-related stress over the past 12 months was relatively mild among those who did not show up for the exam and

Table 1   Pearson Product–Moment Coefficients of Correlation Between Stressors Due to Academic Work, Family, Finance, and One's Own Body and Related Efforts to Cope with These Stressors Among Students 1 Week Ahead of Major Exam

Target for efforts to cope	Stressor			
	Work	Family	Finance	Body
Work	.74***	−.04	.25**	.41***
Family	.07	.62***	.29**	.21*
Finance	.31***	.23**	.80***	.29**
One's own body	.26**	.03	.16	.79***

*$p < .05$. **$p < .01$. ***$p < .001$.

those who failed as compared with the more successful students, $F(4, 76) = 3.85$, $p < .007$. A corresponding group difference was also found for scores on efforts invested to cope with work-related stressors, $F(4, 75) = 2.98$, $p < .024$. Stressors due to other sources, and the related effort, did not distinguish between the participant groups.

The differences between the five participant groups were even greater in scores related to the penultimate week before the exam. Again, work-related stress, $F(4, 71) = 4.70$, $p < .02$, and effort invested to cope with this academic stress, $F(4, 71) = 3.22$, $p < .017$, were high among successful students. In addition, group differences were also significant for scores on efforts to cope with stressors attributed to one's own body, probably symptoms of fear, $F(4, 71) = 3.87$, $p < .007$, with only mild effort being displayed in relation to this stressor by those students who failed. Scores on the pleasant emotion termed *provocativeness* or *as-if anger* (bloodymindedness; cf. the German term *schadenfreude*; implying the paratelic and negativistic states) was significantly higher among students who ended up being nonsuccessful, $F(4, 71) = 3.21$, $p < .018$.

Results from multivariate discriminant classifications of students across the five academic performance groups by scores on stressors, effort, and prevailing emotions over the past 12 months successfully identified 76.9% of the participants. The discriminant function showed that successful students were characterized by high scores on work-related stress, $F(1, 74) = 8.29$, $p < .005$, and high levels of effort invested to cope with stress due to this academic work stressor, $F(1, 74) = 5.78$, $p < .019$.

A corresponding discriminant function was based on scores for the past 7 days just 1 week ahead of the impending exam. In this case, 78.2% of participants were correctly classified across the five performance groups on the basis of a discriminant function where successful students were characterized by high scores on effort to cope with one's own body as a source of stress, $F(1, 74) = 7.32$, $p < .009$, as well as by the experience of high work stress, $F(1, 74) = 6.52$, $p < .013$, and related effort to cope, $F(1, 74) = 7.00$, $p < .010$. Obviously, performance-related anxiety provoked more and more bodily symptoms that had to be dealt with on top of the academic work needed over the days before the exam. Those who were able to exert effort to cope with this stressor of bodily origin, probably related to anxiety and fatigue, were more likely to be among the successful students. Scores on two emotion items loaded on the discriminant function: Students who failed to experience anxiety just before the exam tended to be less successful on the exam, $F(1, 74) = 3.89$, $p < .052$, as was also the case for students who reported relatively high levels of excitement just before the exam, $F(1, 74) = 3.86$, $p < .059$.

CONCLUSION

The results from these two studies support the assumption of a close association between magnitude of perceived stress and amount of effort to cope with the stressor. They also suggest that these associations are domain-specific in the sense that stressors due to, for example, finance fail to provoke effort to cope with academic achievement. Moreover, both studies support the assumption that a major predictor of good performance is the exertion of effort to cope with the stressor.

Findings from the two studies had a different time span for assessments over the past 7 days where items were scored between 2 and 4 weeks ahead of the exam in Study 1 and between 1 and 2 weeks ahead of the exam in Study 2. This difference may explain why ability to cope with one's own body as a major stressor was predictive of performance in the second study, whereas specific emotions such as sullenness and guilt were more sensitive predictors in Study 1. Fear of poor academic performance caused more and more psychobiological turmoil as students approached the day of the exam: Several bodily symptoms are well-established diagnostic criteria of anxiety (e.g., pounding heart, hot spells, tremor, sweating, breathlessness, etc.; see American Psychiatric Association, 1994).

In short, it turned out to be a promising sign of good performance for the individual to evaluate the stressor as high and to exert a corresponding amount of effort to cope over the time of preparation for the exam. Poor performance related to low effort, and these students appeared to pay a double price in that they also reported more tension-stress, particularly in the form of sullenness and guilt. When the time of the exam came very close, tension-stress in the form of anxiety (reflecting the telic state of goal-directedness) was on the average a promising sign, whereas paratelic excitement (indicating the paratelic state of playfulness) predicted poor performance. Coping strategies are likely to be very different for individuals in the telic–conformist (anxiety) and in the paratelic–negativistic (sullenness) states. In this way, strategy as well as intensity of the exertion of effort appeared to be important for successful performance. High effort was predictive of good performance in the long as well as short time spans, and low tension-stress correlated with high effort and excellence when there were still several weeks to the examination. Closer to the examination, the exertion of high effort continued to be predictive of excellence, whereas emotional turmoil in the form of anxiety appeared to be an unavoidable price to pay for the remaining days among students who performed well.

REFERENCES

American Psychiatric Association (1994). *Diagnostic and statistical manual of mental disorders* (4th ed.). Washington, DC: Author.

Barratt, E. S. (1965). Factor analysis of some psychometric measures of impulsiveness and anxiety. *Psychological Reports, 16,* 547–554.

Cacioppo, J. T., & Petty, R. E. (1982). The need for cognition. *Journal of Personality and Social Psychology, 42,* 116–131.

Cannon, W. B. (1927). The James-Lange theory of emotions: A critical examination and an alternative. *American Journal of Psychology, 39,* 106–124.

Duffy, E. (1957). The psychological significance of the concept of "arousal" or "activation." *Psychological Review, 64*, 265–275.

Folkman, S., & Lazarus, R. S. (1985). If it changes it must be a process: Study of emotion and coping during three stages of a college exam. *Journal of Personality and Social Psychology, 48*, 150–170.

Hebb, D. O. (1955). Drives and the C.N.S. (Conceptual Nervous System). *Psychological Review, 62*, 243–254.

Hockey, G. R. J., Gaillard, A. W. K., & Coles, M. G. G. (1986). *Energetics and human information processing*. Dordrecht, The Netherlands: Nijhoff.

Lazarus, R. S., & Folkman, S. (1984). *Stress, appraisal and coping*. New York: Springer Verlag.

Light, K. C. (1985). Cardiovascular and renal responses to competitive mental challenges. In J. F. Orlbeke, G. Mulder, & L. P. J. van Doornen (Eds.), *Psychophysiology of cardiovascular control* (pp. 683–701). New York: Plenum Press.

Obrist, P. A. (1981). *Cardiovascular psychophysiology: A perspective*. New York: Plenum Press.

Strømme, S. B., Wikeby, P. C., Blix, A. S., & Ursin, H. (1978). Additional heart rate. In H. Ursin, E. Baade & S. Levine (Eds.), *Psychobiology of stress: A study of coping men* (pp. 83–89). Academic Press: New York.

Svebak, S. (1988). *Anstrengelse lønner seg: Motivasjon og karakterer til grunnfagseksamen i psykologi* [The payoff of effort: Motivation and marks in the introductory psychology exam] (Monograph No. 7). Bergen, Norway: UNIBUT.

Svebak, S. (1991). The role of effort in stress and emotion. In C. D. Spielberger, I. G. Sarason, Z. Kulcsar, & G. V. Heck (Eds.), *Stress and emotion* (Vol. 14, pp. 121–134). Washington, DC: Hemisphere.

Svebak, S. (1993). The development of the Tension and Effort Stress Inventory (TESI). In J. H. Kerr, S. Murgatroyd, & M. J. Apter (Eds.), *Advances in reversal theory* (pp. 189–204). Amsterdam: Zwets & Zeitlinger.

Ursin, H., & Murison, R. C. (1983). The stress concept. In H. Ursin & R. C. Murison (Eds.), *Biological and psychological basis of psychosomatic disease* (pp. 7–13). London: Pergamon Press.

5

Back Pain and Work Stress

Sven Svebak, Reidar Mykletun, and Edvin Bru

The phenomenological orientation in reversal theory to the study of motivation and emotion makes it of particular relevance for research on psychogenic factors in musculoskeletal complaints. The Tension and Effort Stress Inventory (TESI) was developed to assess amount of effort-stress and tension-stress as defined in reversal theory. This inventory is briefly described. Results from two studies of musculoskeletal pain in the neck, shoulders, and lower back are described. Both involved female employees (bank personnel and hospital staff, respectively) who completed both the TESI and standardized surveys of musculoskeletal pain. One consistent pattern of findings indicated that anxiety and anger may be less involved in back pain than has been assumed in previous research. However, resentment and guilt, two transactional emotions that involve the sympathy mode, appeared to be particularly involved in neck and shoulder pain. In contrast, results support the trend in previous research that shows that dysphoric mood (tension-stress) is not greatly involved in lower back pain. Results from an intervention study are also summarized to support the assumption of a causal role for metamotivational modes and tension-stress in neck and shoulder pain and effort-stress in lower back pain.

There are at least two good reasons to study musculoskeletal tension and pain from the perspective of reversal theory. First, the activity patterns of the skeletal muscles are controlled by the central nervous system in a way that permits partial voluntary control. This arrangement is located in the so-called monosynaptic pyramidal pathways from the motor and sensory sections of the cerebral cortex to the skeletal muscles. This is not to downplay the significance of those pathways for skeletal motor control that are not under voluntary control, the extremely complex extrapyramidal pathways to the skeletal muscles,

The research reviewed in this chapter was supported by grants from the Norwegian Research Counsel Medical Research Branch and sources at the University of Bergen, Norway.

such as the nerve fibers of the reticulospinal tract. A major function of these latter pathways is to provide a concerted action of background muscle tension throughout the skeletal muscles. The aim of this function is to ensure the automatic modulation of adequate body posture when full attention is required by intellectual work, artistic performance, sports, or skilled performance at work. The pyramidal pathway is the only motor system that can be under direct conscious control. The most obvious opposite case is the autonomic nervous system, so named because it is not under conscious control, meaning that people are not able to adjust functions such as blood pressure and gastric secretion in any direct way by volition.

The second reason for studying musculoskeletal tension and pain from the reversal theory perspective is the sophisticated phenomenological analysis of motivation and emotion provided in reversal theory. The musculoskeletal system is closely associated with such processes, both in body posture, movement, and work output as well as in expressive display and control of emotional states. Reversal theory might therefore open up new approaches to research in musculoskeletal tension and pain.

The focus in this chapter is on musculoskeletal pain rather than on muscle tension. Pain is always a subjective experience attributed to one's own body and one that signals malfunction or risk of malfunction or tissue damage. Pain is therefore an important signal to help the individual take action for self-protection. This function is particularly evident in the rare case when an individual is born without the capacity for nociception; this condition can be life-threatening because of the absence of signals such as pain behavior, including crying, that help parents take action on behalf of a small child (Sternbach, 1968).

The sources of musculoskeletal pain are various, and a full account is beyond the scope of this chapter. Some of them reflect tissue damage of the contractile segment or the tendons of the muscle, whereas others involve circulatory dysfunctions such as ischemia or inflammatory processes related to tissue damage of the muscle itself or of nerves that communicate with skeletal muscles. Skeletal malfunction and spinal disk prolapse are other sources of pain, and some instances of musculoskeletal pain are of unknown origin and may involve dysfunctions of the central nervous system itself (Cervero & Laird, 1991).

Several years ago, Borchrevink, Brekke, and Øgar (1980) reported that 20% of patients treated by general practitioners in Norway suffered from musculoskeletal complaints. They also estimated that approximately 30% of time lost through sick leave was due to such complaints where they involved pain. Several more recent studies have confirmed these findings from industrialized societies (Lee, Helewa, Smythe, Bombardier, & Goldsmith, 1985; Tellnes, 1989; Westgaard & Aaras, 1984).

Most of the musculoskeletal research in recent years has focused on lower back pain. A major finding is that men appear to have more frequent episodes of lower back pain than do women, whereas women tend to report pain in neck and shoulders more frequently than do men (Lee et al., 1985: Ursin, Endresen, & Ursin, 1988). General practitioners tend to perceive lower back pain as one of the most frustrating and unrewarding conditions to manage, partly because of inadequate diagnostic methods and training (Deyo, Cherkin, Conrad, & Volinn, 1991) and partly because of the negative attitudes that develop among the junior primary care doctors during their orthopaedic training (Skelton, Murphy, Murphy, & O'Dowd, 1995). Skelton et al. reported seven different dimensions that general practitioners use to distinguish among patients with lower back pain in order to decide how to treat them: the patient's psychological constitution, clinical condition, approach to management, help-seeking behavior, social class, sex, and occupation. All these traditional dimensions are of obvious relevance and may help in the design of treatment. However, a few recent studies of back pain, involving the neck and shoulders as well as the lower back, have adopted a new assessment methodology developed within reversal theory. Findings from these studies offer new insight into the psychological characteristics of patients with back pain, and they are reviewed in this chapter.

THE TENSION AND EFFORT STRESS INVENTORY

The TESI is a one-page survey that reflects the reversal theory analysis of stress. It is divided into three sections to measure the experience of (a) sources of stress, (b) related coping efforts, and (c) a set of eight pleasant and eight unpleasant moods or emotions. More specifically, the first section provides four items on the experience of sources of stress (pressure, stress, challenge, or demand) over the past 30 days as related to work, family, finance, and the person's own body, respectively. The second section consists of four items (work, family, finance, own body) that ask about the degree of effort "that you have put up over the last thirty days to cope with pressure etc. from [the four domains of life stress reflected in the four items]." This section, therefore, provides estimates of the degree of effort-stress (as defined in Chapter 2 and in Apter & Svebak, 1989).

Tension-stress is reflected in the third section of the TESI where eight items assess degree of unpleasant moods or emotions over the past 30 days: anxiety, boredom, anger, sullenness, humiliation, shame, resentment, and guilt. Another eight items in this section assess the range of pleasant emotional experiences or moods (relaxation, excitement, placidity, provocativeness, pride, modesty, gratitude, and virtue; see also Chapters 1 and 2). All items are scored in terms of a 7-point scale (1 = *no pressure, effort, or emotional experience*; 7 = *very much*). The TESI itself as well as suggestions for scoring it have been published elsewhere (Svebak, 1993).

The TESI would be of no use in back pain research without the availability of valid methods for the measurement of back pain. Our studies to be reported here made use of a Standardized Nordic Questionnaire (SNQ) for the analysis of musculoskeletal symptoms (due to Kourinka et al., 1987). This survey measure includes a section on symptoms in the neck, shoulders, and lower back with estimates for the past 12 months and for the past 7 days. Information from this section was combined with information on sick leave as well as number of complaint periods over the past 6 months to obtain an index of chronic back pain.

THE RELATION BETWEEN MUSCLE PAIN AND TENSION

Anxiety has been the most frequently investigated emotion related to musculo-skeletal pain. There are probably two major reasons for this interest in anxiety. First, Malmo (1975) conducted a series of studies on associations between anxiety and the tensing of skeletal muscles during perceptual motor task performance. He noted that electromyographic indications of increasing muscle tension occurred in muscles that were not called on by the extrinsic nature of the task (e.g., performance of a tracking task by use of the dominant hand and elevated muscle tension in the nondominant hand). This tendency was more marked in anxious participants. The second hypothesis is that of a close if not linear association between levels of muscle tension and risk of muscle pain. Although Malmo provided support for this idea for some samples of participants under some circumstances, results from several recent electromyographic studies indicate no more than a weak association between levels of muscle tension and levels of muscle pain (e.g., Svebak, Anjia, & Kårstad, 1993).

Furthermore, Schmidt and Wallace (1982) concluded that the emotional states of anger and aggression are not significantly implicated in lower back pain. Likewise, Love and Peck (1987) found little support in Minnesota Multiphasic Personality Inventory studies for the assumption of a causal psychogenic factor in lower back pain (see also Bradley, Prokop, Margolis & Gentry, 1978; Schmidt & Arntz, 1987). Two limitations are obvious in these previous studies of personality factors related to motivation and emotion in musculoskeletal pain: First, most of the studies on pain have looked specifically at pain in the lower back. Second, previous studies have assessed a very limited range of unpleasant emotions, especially anxiety and anger. Depression has also been studied in some cases, but they may not qualify as studies of any particular emotional experience because depression can be colored by different emotional qualities such as anxiety, boredom, guilt, or humiliation. For these reasons, it was felt that a more inclusive approach, guided by reversal theory and using methods for the assessment of a wider range of muscle pain and of emotions or moods, might provide a more complete and accurate test of possible associations between psychological states and stress-related musculoskeletal pain.

A STUDY OF BANK EMPLOYEES

Bru, Mykletun, and Svebak (1994) reported data that showed the importance of distinguishing between three body areas of musculoskeletal pain: the neck and shoulders, the lower back, and the extremities, respectively. The SNQ, which was used in this study (as described above), has a diagrammatic guide to the distinction between these areas of the body. In the first TESI-based study, 96 female bank employees were recruited on the basis of their responses to the SNQ (Svebak, Ursin, Endresen, Hjelmen, & Apter, 1991). They presented a distribution from mild to severe symptoms of musculoskeletal pain in one or more of the areas defined according to hatched segments in a figure of the body in the SNQ, defined as the neck, shoulders, and lower back, respectively. Their mean age was 32.2 (range = 20–62), and their mean working hours per week were 36.1 (range = 8–50; for further details, see Svebak et al., 1991).

All participants volunteered for the study after having completed a first-stage survey submitted to 350 employees in the company. Of the 60% who completed the initial survey, 70% reported musculoskeletal complaints over the previous month. All who participated in the second stage presented at least mild pain in one of the areas of the back, and all were examined by a rheumatologist to exclude cases of fibromyalgia, damage due to accidents, or previous hospitalization for back trouble due to neurological or osteological diseases.

The survey measures (SNQ, TESI) were used as part of a more extensive set of questionnaires; participants completed all questionnaires during a visit to the medical care unit of the company. Participants were all informed that the aim of the survey was to improve the empirical basis for intervention procedures in the treatment of back complaints.

Results from correlational analyses of bivariate associations between emotions and back pain scores yielded surprising findings. Among the unpleasant emotions, anxiety was not significantly associated with pain scores from any area of the back, and neither were scores on boredom and sullenness. However, anger did show some association with scores on pain in neck and shoulders (rs = .26 and 29, respectively, $p < .04$). Interestingly, unpleasant emotions due to failure to cope with interpersonal relations (humiliation, shame, resentment, and guilt, the so-called transactional emotions; see Apter, 1988) were more associated with pain in the back. For example, scores on resentment explained almost 50% of the variance in overall back pain scores, this being essentially due to high coefficients of correlation with scores for the neck and shoulder. A similar pattern of associations was found for scores on guilt (see Table 1). Scores on humiliation and shame were associated with pain from the shoulder area ($p < .05$).

This sample revealed only two significant correlations between back pain scores and pleasant emotional states. One of these was a negative association for relaxation with pain in shoulders over the past week ($r = -0.28$, $p < .04$), and the other revealed a positive association for pride with pain in the shoulders over the past year ($r = 0.37$, $p < .01$). The former pain may reflect mild, but enduring, activation of the shoulder muscles (trapezius, deltoid, etc.), whereas the latter pain may reflect a postural component of pride where the upper body is kept more erect and the shoulders retracted when experiencing pride (see the term *soldier's posture*, proposed by Heckscher, 1938). Keeping in mind the point made above that there is only a loose association between muscle tension

Table 1   Pearson Product–Moment Correlations Between
Scores for Back Complaints Over the Past Year and Scores
for the Experience of Unpleasant Emotions or Moods
in Transactions with Others

	Complaint			
Emotion	Neck	Shoulders	Lower back	Total
Humiliation	0.04	0.24†	0.17	0.22†
Shame	0.13	0.33†	0.11	0.23†
Resentment	0.48*	0.55**	0.35*	0.68**
Guilt	0.30*	0.42*	0.25†	0.50*

*$p < .01$, two-tailed. **$p < .001$. $^{\dagger}p < .05$, one-tailed.

and pain, another possible mechanism might be that of ischemia due to sympathetic nerve influences on vessels that shunt blood through the skeletal muscles. Ischemia may be induced in the neck and shoulder muscles with enduring and moderate muscle tension caused by anger, resentment, and guilt.

The pattern of findings from this study, then, indicates a risk of neck and shoulder pain in particular among participants dominated by the telic and negativistic modes (and experiencing anger frequently), the sympathy and autic or alloic modes (frequently experiencing resentment and guilt, respectively), or the mastery and autic modes (experiencing pride frequently; see Chapter 1).

Another line of TESI scores reflected the perceived amount of exposure to stressors and related efforts to cope (effort-stress). Surprisingly weak associations were found generally, and the only significant correlation that emerged was that between neck pain and effort invested to cope with stressors due to work ($r = 0.22$, $p < .05$). Stressors and related efforts attributed to family and finance were unrelated to pain scores. In contrast, scores on stressors and related efforts to cope that were attributed to one's own body were consistently high with pain in neck ($p < .001$) and shoulders, as well as the lower back ($p < .01$). This means that, phenomenologically, the body was perceived as the major source of stressors and as the greatest challenge in terms of efforts to cope in participants with back pain. Consequently, back pain may well be the result of extrinsic ergonomic or emotional load, but the pain was perceived by participants as the major challenge in coping with life stress. In this way, body complaints may be caused by extrinsic stressors and then themselves become stressors, thus triggering a vicious circle of events.

A STUDY OF FEMALE HOSPITAL STAFF

The same survey measures as those used in the preceding study were later administered to female hospital staff in different departments at a regional hospital in Norway (Bru, Mykletun, & Svebak, 1994). In this study, Bru et al. also included a more focused scale on how musculoskeletal pain might interfere with the performance of daily activities (see Westgaard & Jansen, 1992, for details on this scale, including data on reliability and validity). The rate of participation in this study was 85% and resulted in a sample of 547 female staff after exclusion of 39 participants (owing to rheumatoid arthritis, Bechterew's disease, epilepsy, previous surgery to the spine, osteoporosis, breast cancer, fibromyalgia, and pregnancy).

The survey in this study was administered during working hours, with those on day shift completing the forms during a visit to the health care unit and those working in the evening or at night responding on the ward. In all cases, respondents were left undisturbed, but a research assistant was always present to ensure standardized conditions and the clarification of questions whenever they were raised (for further methodological details, see Bru et al., 1994).

Seventy-seven percent of the sample reported musculoskeletal complaints from the neck, shoulders, or lower back over the previous 12 months. Complaints were more frequent in connection with the lower back (55%) than the neck (49%) and the shoulders (42%). Between 5% and 10% reported severe pain, whereas the rest of the sample reported mild to moderate levels of back pain.

The TESI scores on work-related stress and degree of effort were generally in the medium range. Emotion scores were in the low to medium range on the average, and pleasant emotions were somewhat more prevalent than unpleasant ones. Highest mean emotion scores were found for the experience of gratitude and placidity (indicating relatively successful coping in the metamotivational modes of sympathy–autic and telic–negativistic, respectively). The most prevalent unpleasant emotions were anger and anxiety (reflecting poor coping within the telic–negativistic and telic–conformist modes, respectively).

Significantly high positive correlations were found between scores on overall stress and degree of effort ($r = .83$, $p < .0001$), as well as between work-specific stress and efforts ($r = .79$, $p < .0001$). Generally, overall tension-stress scores correlated significantly with total stress and degree of effort ($rs = .49$ and .46, respectively) and with work-specific sources of stress and degree of effort ($rs = .37$ and .34, respectively; all coefficients were significant beyond the .01 level). Interestingly, overall scores on pleasant emotions were unrelated to back pain, whereas overall tension-stress scores yielded significant positive coefficients with neck pain ($r = .26$), shoulder pain ($r = .17$), and pain in the lower back ($r = .14$). Similar ranges of correlations were found for scores on stress and degree of effort, and all coefficients were significant at the 1% level (two-tailed; $N = 547$).

A more detailed approach to the association between tension-stress and back pain looked at particular types of tension-stress, that is, different unpleasant emotions. Generally, coefficients of correlation were low (from .05 to .23). Nonsignificant relations were found for the association of shoulder pain with

Table 2   Spearman Product–Moment Coefficients
of Correlation Between Pain in the Neck, Shoulders,
and Lower Back with the Experience of Eight Dysphoric
Emotions (Tension-Stress) Among Midwives

		Complaint	
Emotion	Neck	Shoulders	Lower Back
Anxiety	0.34[t]	0.44[t]	−0.01
Boredom	0.30*	0.45*	−0.17
Anger	0.38*	0.41*	−0.13
Sullenness	0.45*	0.61*	−0.13
Humiliation	0.41*	0.34[t]	0.04
Shame	0.22	0.46*	0.06
Resentment	0.23	0.47*	−0.07
Guilt	0.50*	0.59*	0.21

*$p < .01$, two-tailed. [t]$p < .05$, one-tailed.

shame and sullenness and for the association of lower back pain with anxiety and boredom, whereas scores on neck pain were significantly associated with all the unpleasant emotions. A distinction was made here between eight subsamples, to reflect the differences between staff working in departments with varying degrees of ergonomic load (relatively high in orthopaedic and internal medicine wards) and emotional load (relatively high among midwives). Interestingly, the subsample assumed to be exposed to the highest levels of emotional load (midwives, $n = 37$) also yielded the highest correlations for tension-stress with back pain (see Table 2). The highest coefficients were found with these participants for sullenness and guilt with pain in the shoulders (indicating poor coping in the paratelic–negativistic and sympathy–alloic modes, respectively). Also, consistently nonsignificant coefficients of correlation were found in this group for lower back pain with tension-stress.

A final test involved the use of simultaneous multiple regression (path analysis) on these data. This approach tested the idea of a mediating effect of tension-stress (dysphoria) and a moderating effect of good moods (euphoria) on the relation between work-stress and overall back pain as well as on work-related efforts and overall back pain. Results from the latter analysis are illustrated in Figure 1. They support the idea that effort-stress increases the risk of back pain, that tension-stress is a mediator of this risk, and that the experience of good moods (absence of tension-stress) when expending effort moderates the risk of back pain due to effort-stress. The effect of perceived stress on back pain was kept constant in these path analyses and meant that relations illustrated in Figure 1 were free from confounding effects of other variables in the TESI.

Apter and Svebak (1989; see also Chapter 2) argued that the perception of stressors involves the induction of tension-stress unless effort-stress is invested to

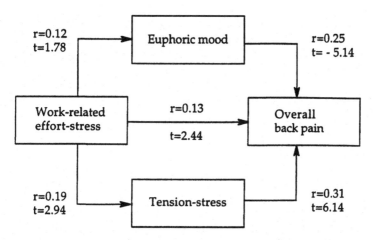

Figure 1 A test of the assumption of a direct effect of work-related effort-stress (efforts invested to cope with stress at work) on overall back pain and the mediating effect of tension-stress (dysphoric moods) as well as the moderating effect of pleasant emotions (euphoric moods). Partial correlations and t scores are given. Note the negative t score for the relation between euphoric moods and back pain (support of moderating effect of pleasant emotions) and the positive t score for the relation between dysphoric moods and back pain (support of a mediating effect of tension-stress on back pain). All t scores are statistically significant; $N = 547$.

overcome the tension-stress. They also argued that the worst possible outcome in coping with stressors is the expenditure of high effort without successful coping, which results in the additional burden of experiencing tension-stress. These effects are strongly supported in the direct and mediating effects presented in Figure 1. Moreover, Apter and Svebak argued that the expenditure of effort-stress that successfully overcomes tension-stress may have beneficial effects on health. This argument was also supported by the highly significant mediating effect shown in the upper section of Figure 1. Separate analyses were performed for the neck, shoulder, and lower back pain scores, and they paralleled the patterns shown in Figure 1 except for weaker coefficients and t scores when the model was applied to lower back pain than when applied to neck and shoulder pain.

Taken together, these findings lend support for a role for effort-stress as well as for tension-stress in back pain, and for tension-stress in neck and shoulder pain in particular. However, these studies were all correlational. Therefore, Bru, Mykletun, Berge, and Svebak (1994) conducted an intervention program with a sample of 168 participants from the largest sample of hospital staff. Three treatment programs were offered: (a) cognitive intervention to improve communication skills and ways of coping with the work environment, including occupational demands and emotional load; (b) muscular relaxation with a focus on the procedure developed by Jacobson (1938), and (c) a combination of the cognitive and relaxation procedures for stress management. Participants were randomly assigned to the three intervention procedures or to a fourth group defined as a waiting-list control group. Results supported the conclusion that cognitive and combined procedures were superior in reducing pain in the neck and shoulders, whereas relaxation was superior in the treatment of lower back pain. These conclusions were also supported by reports on pain at a 4-month follow-up (see Bru, Mykletun, Berge, & Svebak, 1994, for details). These findings indicate a predominantly causal role for tension-stress in neck and shoulder pain and for effort-stress in lower back pain.

CONCLUSION

New insight on back pain has been achieved from research using a survey measure derived from reversal theory. One pattern of findings from these studies underlined the importance of a distinction between pain in the neck and shoulders and pain in the lower back. Tension-stress in the form of resentment and guilt was particularly prevalent among female employees, indicating a particular role for the so-called sympathy mode in lack of coping with interpersonal relations at work. A study of hospital staff provided support for the argument that effort-stress plus tension-stress would be the worst possible psychogenic risk for the development of bodily complaints, and the mediating role for tension-stress with effort-stress was particularly marked for pain in the neck and shoulders. A causal role was indicated for tension-stress in that an intervention with a focus on improvement of competence in interpersonal relations proved superior to relaxation training in reducing neck and shoulder pain, whereas relaxation training was superior in reducing lower back pain.

Using studies of musculoskeletal pain in the neck, shoulders, and lower back, this chapter has explored the physical repercussions of anxiety and anger as well as other emotions. Certainly, reasons for studying musculoskeletal tension and pain from the perspective of reversal theory have been validated by the studies explored here.

REFERENCES

Apter, M. J. (1988). Reversal theory as a theory of the emotions. In M. J. Apter, J. H. Kerr, & M. P. Cowles (Eds.), *Progress in reversal theory: Vol. 51. Advances in psychology* (pp. 43–62). Amsterdam: North-Holland/Elsevier.

Apter, M. J., & Svebak, S. (1989). Stress from the reversal theory perspective. In C. D. Spielberger, I. G. Sarason, & J. Strelau (Eds.), *Stress and emotion* (Vol. 12, pp 39–52). Washington, DC: Hemisphere.

Borchrevink, C. F., Brekke, T. H., & Øgar, B. (1980). Musculo-skeletal illness in general practice. *Tidsskrift for Den Norske Laegeforening (Journal of the Norwegian Medical Association), 100,* 439–445.

Bradley, L. A., Prokop, C. K., Margolis, R., & Gentry, W. D. (1978). Multivariate analyses of the MMPI profiles of low back pain patients. *Journal of Behavioral Medicine, 3,* 253–272.

Bru, E., Mykletun, R. J., Berge, W. T., & Svebak, S. (1994). Effects of different psychological interventions on neck, shoulder and low back pain in female hospital staff. *Psychology and Health, 9,* 371–382.

Bru, E., Mykletun, R. J., & Svebak, S. (1994). Assessment of musculoskeletal and other health complaints in female hospital staff. *Applied Ergonomics, 25,* 101–105.

Bru, E., Mykletun, R. J., & Svebak, S. (1997). Back pain, dysphoric versus euphoric moods and the experience of stress and efforts in female hospital staff. *Personality and Individual Differences,* in press.

Cervero, F., & Laird, J. M. A. (1991). One pain or many pains? A new look at pain mechanisms. *News in Physiological Sciences, 6,* 268–273.

Deyo, R. A., Cherkin, D., Conrad, D., & Volinn, E. (1991). Cost, controversy, crisis: Low back pain and the health of the public. *Annual Review of Public Health, 12,* 141–156.

Heckscher, H. (1938). Neurosis cordis et respirationis [Heart neurosis and respiration]. *Ugeskrift for Leger, 100,* 930–937.

Jacobson, E. (1938). *Progressive relaxation* (2nd ed.). Chicago: University of Chicago Press.

Kourinka, I., Jonsson, B., Kilbom, A., Vinterberg, H., Biering-Sørensen, F., Andersson, G., & Jørgensen, K. (1987). Standardised Nordic Questionnaires for the analysis of musculoskeletal symptoms. *Applied Ergonomics, 18,* 233–237.

Lee, P., Helewa, A., Smythe, H. A., Bombardier, C., & Goldsmith, C. H. (1985). Epidemiology of musculoskeletal disorders (complaints) and related disability in Canada. *Journal of Rheumatology, 12,* 1169–1173.

Love, A. W., & Peck, C. L. (1987). The MMPI and psychological factors in chronic low back pain: A review. *Pain, 28,* 1–12.

Malmo, R. B. (1975). *On emotions, needs, and our archaic brain.* New York: Holt, Rinehart & Winston.

Schmidt, A. J. M., & Arntz, A. (1987). Psychological research and chronic low back pain: A stand-still or breakthrough? *Social Sciences in Medicine, 25,* 1095–1104.

Schmidt, J. P., & Wallace, R. W. (1982). Factorial analysis of the MMPI profiles of low back pain patients. *Journal of Personality Assessment, 46,* 366–369.

Skelton, A. M., Murphy, E. A., Murphy, R. J. L., & O'Dowd, T. C. (1995). General practitioner perceptions of low back pain patients. *Family Practice, 12,* 44–48.

Svebak, S. (1993). The development of the tension and effort stress inventory (TESI). In J. H. Kerr, S. Murgatroyd, & M. J. Apter (Eds.), *Advances in reversal theory* (pp. 189–204). Amsterdam: Swets & Zeitlinger.

Svebak, S., Anjia, R., & Kårstad, S. I. (1993). Task-induced electromyographic activation in fibromyalgia subjects and controls. *Scandinavian Journal of Rheumatology, 22,* 124–130.

Svebak, S., Ursin, H., Endresen, I., Hjelmen, A. M., & Apter, M. J. (1991). Back pain and the experience of stress, efforts and moods. *Psychology and Health, 5,* 307–314.

Tellnes, G. (1989). Days lost by sickness certification. *Scandinavian Journal of Primary Health Care, 7,* 245–251.

Ursin, H., Endresen, I. M., & Ursin, G. (1988). Psychological factors and self-reports of muscle pain. *European Journal of Applied Physiology, 57,* 282–290.

Westgaard, R. H., & Aaras, A. (1984). Postural muscle strain as a causal factor in the development of musculo-skeletal illness. *Applied Ergonomics, 15,* 162–174.

Westgaard, R. H., & Jensen, T. (1992). Individual and work-related factors associated with symptoms of musculoskeletal complaints. I: A quantitative registration system. *British Journal of Industrial Medicine, 49,* 147–153.

6

The Psychobiology
of Telic Dominance and Stress

Rod A. Martin and Sven Svebak

Because low levels of felt arousal are preferred in the telic state and high arousal levels are preferred in the paratelic state, it has been proposed that telic-dominant individuals tend to cope with threat and everyday hassles in ways that are different from paratelic-dominant individuals. This personality difference may also involve physiological differences and, therefore, represent different levels of risk for somatic complaints and diseases. Results from psychophysiological laboratory studies and immune-related studies of stressful life events are reviewed in this chapter as they relate to the distinction between telic and paratelic dominance. The pattern of findings from these studies suggests that paratelic-dominant individuals respond with low tension in muscles not called on by extrinsic ergonomic demands, but they respond with high acute-force output in muscles that are called on by the extrinsic nature of motor tasks performed within a threatening context. Their cardiovascular activation is moderate with threat. Conversely, these individuals appear to respond with a reduction of immunoglobulin A (IgA) secretion and elevated secretion of cortisol with the tension of boredom. In contrast, for telic-dominant individuals, unintended muscle tension and cardiovascular response magnitudes appear to be larger and cardiovascular reactivity seems to be mediated by coronary-prone Type A behavior in threatening situations. Successful coping with everyday stressful events seems to result in low cortisol secretion, whereas IgA secretion seems to be positively associated with increased levels of cortisol secretion. Taken together, these findings indicate several psychobiological relations that distinguish between telic- and paratelic-dominant individuals and put them at risk for different health problems.

Several clinical studies have indicated a difference between telic- and paratelic-dominant individuals in the way in which they cope with everyday problems, including frustrations, hassles, threats, and crises. Thus, Baker (1988) showed that telic-dominant individuals would be more likely to appraise everyday bothersome events as threatening and that paratelic-dominant individuals would view such events as challenging. Also, she proposed that telic-dominant individuals would be more likely to report goal-oriented, problem-focused coping strategies, whereas paratelic-dominant individuals would be more likely to report emotion-focused strategies in their responses to everyday hassles.

A study of 15 telic- and 15 paratelic-dominant individuals (Baker, 1988) confirmed the dominance-related difference in perception of life events as threatening versus challenging (29% vs. 39%, respectively among telic-dominant individuals; 9% vs. 59 %, respectively, among paratelic individuals). Furthermore, telic-dominant individuals showed a higher preference for direct action in coping with stress, whereas paratelic-dominant individuals more frequently reported the use of coping styles such as distraction, seeking social support, and leisurely activities. Clinical evidence along the same lines has been published by Murgatroyd (1981).

The purpose of this chapter is to review a series of rigorously controlled laboratory and field studies that complement the clinical investigations of Baker and Murgatroyd (see also Svebak & Stoyva, 1980). These studies all focused on differences between telic- and paratelic-dominant individuals in their ways of coping psychobiologically with potential threats and hassles.

LABORATORY STUDIES

Svebak and his students at the University of Bergen conducted a series of laboratory studies in the 1980s to test the psychophysiological characteristics of telic- and paratelic-dominant participants. These studies have been reviewed in detail elsewhere (Apter, 1989; Apter & Svebak, 1989). Most of them adopted a range of computerized perceptual-motor tasks, such as a car-racing task in which a car could be controlled on video screen by the participant. Designs permitted comparison of psychophysiological response patterns across the telic–paratelic dimension. These response patterns could be compared with the findings reported by Malmo and his associates from mirror-tracking tasks some 30 years earlier (Malmo, 1965).

The modern microprocessor-generated tasks were carefully selected by Svebak to permit experimental manipulation in several ways. Motor response patterns involved only minimal physical workload and very simple movement patterns, such as the tilting of a joystick from one side to the opposite by means of the dominant hand. They could be made more difficult by increasing the speed of the car on the video display. Some experiments involved the threat of electric shock as a consequence of making errors beyond some unspecified level. Ethical considerations required that participants in the latter experiments be taken through an introductory procedure to determine the level of intensity of shock that was perceived as clearly aversive, but not painful. In fact, shocks were never given during task performance and were, therefore, not confounded with quality of task performance. Thus, the manipulation of threat relied completely on the psychological effect of expectancy.

Several physiological parameters were recorded in resting pre- and post-task periods as well as during task performance in these experiments. The parameters included the recording of (a) skeletal muscle tension by use of electromyography from muscles that were involved in the operation of the joystick (active forearm) and muscles not called on directly by the task (passive forearm), (b) cardiovascular activity (heart rate, pulse transit time), (c) respiratory activity (inhalation–exhalation cycle time), and (d) electroencephalographic activity of the brain cortex. Some of the studies involved a distinction between phasic and tonic response changes during task performance. A phasic change is fast, of short duration, and elicited by a particular external influence. A tonic response, in contrast, is slow, of relatively long duration, and occurs for reasons that are not easily referable to any specific extrinsic influence. The presentation that follows concentrates on electromyographic (EMG) and cardiovascular findings from these studies.

EMG RESPONSE PATTERNS

Tonic changes of EMG activity were referred to by Malmo (1965) as the EMG gradient. Typically, a tonic build-up of EMG activity takes place over the course of continuous perceptual-motor task performance or may reach an asymptote of mild tension after a minute or so and returns back to the pretask activity level at the termination of task performance.

Threat of electric shock was manipulated by Svebak, Storfjell, and Dalen (1982) to induce the telic state in randomly recruited participants. On the average, participants were significantly more serious-minded when performing in the shock condition as compared with the no-shock condition. This shift was indicated by scores on the Telic State Measure. Also, threat of shock provoked EMG gradients that were relatively marked compared with those in the no-threat condition.

Extremely dominant telic (serious-minded) and extremely dominant paratelic (playful) individuals were manipulated (Svebak, 1984). The speed of the cars was low in the easy-task version, which was repeated five times with resting periods in between. In contrast, speed was very high in the difficult-task version that was performed only once as the final run. The telic-dominant participants responded with marked EMG gradients in their passive forearms when performing the easy version of this task. This response pattern became less marked with practice. Such gradients were not present in the passive forearm of the paratelic-dominant group, either during the repeated easy task performances or during the very difficult task performance. In contrast, the latter group responded with marked phasic EMG amplitudes of the active forearm. This kind of response occurred with only moderate amplitudes among the telic-dominant participants, and the group difference was particularly marked when performing the very difficult final run. Responses to a state measure confirmed that participants maintained their dominant state in the laboratory situation.

Another extreme group experiment confirmed findings from this study and provided external validity for the psychophysiological laboratory data. This was achieved by the use of structured blind interviews about everyday lifestyles (Svebak & Murgatroyd, 1985). The difference between high and low muscle tension responses found in the laboratory paralleled differences in lifestyles along lines that corresponded well with the defining criteria of telic versus paratelic dominance (see Svebak & Murgatroyd, 1985, for case illustrations of lifestyles).

In a subsequent study, extremely telic- and paratelic-dominant individuals were recruited to a similar laboratory experiment that involved the threat of shock for inferior performance (Svebak, 1986). Again, telic dominance emerged as a psychological characteristic of those who responded with elevations of tension in muscles not directly required for performing the task. This pattern was particularly marked for telic-dominant participants in the threat-of-shock condition (see Figure 1, which also includes data on cardiovascular reactivity). Taken together, these results suggest that telic-dominant individuals experience a higher level of tension, particularly in muscles that are not directly required for task performance, whereas paratelic-dominant individuals seem to display a more task-appropriate allocation of muscle tension. These differences in physi-

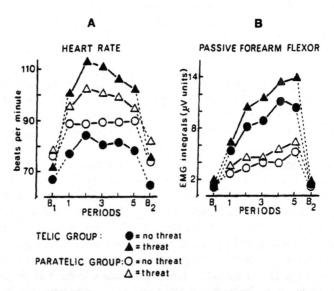

Figure 1 Electromyographic response patterns in the flexor carpi radialis muscle of the passive forearm and cardiovascular response magnitudes in telic- versus paratelic-dominant participants during perceptual motor task performance with and without threat of electric shock for inferior performance. [Adapted from Svebak, S. (1986). Cardiac and somatic activation in the continuous perceptual-motor task: The significance of threat and serious-mindedness. *International Journal of Psychophysiology, 3,* 155–162.]

ological response may occur because telic-dominant individuals appraise such a task as more serious and demanding, whereas paratelic-dominant people approach it in a more playful and less threatened manner. These findings are consistent with the hypothesis that telic-dominant, as compared with paratelic-dominant, individuals are more adversely affected by stress and suggest that they may in turn be more prone to health problems associated with chronic muscle tension.

Kerr and Svebak adopted a very different perspective on musculoskeletal activity patterns by studying the association of telic and paratelic dominance with sport preferences. They reported evidence for a systematic association between telic dominance and preference for endurance sports—long distance running and rowing—whereas preference for explosive sports—baseball, cricket, touch football, downhill skiing, motor racing, and so forth—was predominant among paratelic sport performers (Kerr & Svebak, 1989; Svebak & Kerr, 1989). It is a well-documented fact in sport physiology that these groups of sports reflect the distinction between aerobic and nonaerobic metabolic demands (i.e., the ability of skeletal muscles to develop moderate force for a long time period versus the ability to develop high force that transforms into fatigue quickly). These types of metabolic activity are linked to the distinction between so-called fast- versus slow-twitch muscle fibers, respectively, and the proportional distribution of these fibers is markedly different between skilled performers of endurance and explosive sports. An international champion among endurance sport performers typically has around 80% slow-twitch fibers in the leg gastrocnemius muscle, and the opposite pattern is found in biopsies from elite performers of explosive sports where around 80% of the fibers in this muscle are fast twitch. These differences are essentially genetically defined (Fox, 1984).

From these studies, the idea emerged that the EMG gradient among telic-dominant individuals may have a genetic foundation. Therefore, a biopsy study was conducted to relate the proportion of slow-twitch fibers to the tendency for developing marked EMG gradients when performing perceptual-motor tasks in the laboratory. Results confirmed the association between marked EMG gradients and a predominance of slow-twitch fibers (Svebak et al., 1993). All these findings, taken together, suggest a genetic basis for telic as well as paratelic dominance and that this basis involves a difference in the composition of skeletal muscles.

This is not to say that individuals who are prone to respond with elevated muscle tension in threatening situations will necessarily be at high risk of developing muscle pain. Recent studies have indicated that psychogenic factors can be involved in muscle pain by means of other mechanisms than those related directly to muscle tension. Muscles with a predominance of slow-twitch fibers are genetically prepared for the induction of moderate work output over long time periods, and tension levels seen in passive muscles during perceptual-motor task performance and in other activities may therefore be performed without a high risk of fatigue and related pain. However, some individuals may have acquired a telic-dominant lifestyle throughout childhood and adolescence, and this lifestyle may in some cases fail to match the genetically given talents of their skeletal muscles. In such cases when the brain activates neural pathways to skeletal muscle activation and the individual is in the telic mode, moderate levels of enduring muscle tension may not be tolerated in the muscle owing to a predominance of fast-twitch fibers. A resulting outcome may be pain in this particular constellation of psychological and biological characteristics. Ischemia (blood supply short of actual metabolic demands) may also cause pain. Emotions influence cardiovascular functions in several ways, and many of them are not yet well understood. It has been shown that resentment and guilt seem to be particularly involved in neck and shoulder pain (Svebak, Ursin, Endresen, Hjelmen, & Apter, 1991; see also Chapter 5). These findings indicate that for some types of muscle pain, other dominant modes, such as the sympathy mode, rather than telic dominance, may be involved in risk of pain in the neck and shoulders.

CARDIOVASCULAR RESPONSE PATTERNS

Svebak et al. (1982) recorded heart rate in addition to EMG response in their study of the motivational consequences of the threat versus no-threat manipulation. The typical pattern for heart rate in perceptual-motor task performance with minimal physical workload is an early peak that may decline somewhat over the rest of the task performance and then return to the prebaseline level when the task is over. Overall, this elevation was significantly higher within the threat condition than it was in the no-threat condition. In the threat condition, heart rate increased more than 20 beats per minute above baseline, whereas the increase was only around 8 beats per minute on average without threat. A response magnitude of 20 beats per minute observed in the psychophysiological laboratory is considered quite substantial. In fact, a response magnitude of this size might be of some clinical relevance for risk of future cardiac events in some individuals.

A later study by Svebak (1986) involved a comparison of extremely dominant telic and paratelic participants in the threat and no-threat conditions. Heart rate elevations were particularly marked among the telic-dominant participants in the threat condition, but were relatively low in the no-threat condition. The paratelic-dominant individuals reflected the same trend, but their heart rates fell between those of the telic-dominant participants. It is worth pointing out that the magnitude of cardiac responses in task performance with threat was on average more than 40 beats per minute among the telic-dominant individuals (see Figure 1).

Svebak and Apter (1984) reported a nonsignificant relationship between telic dominance and the so-called coronary-prone Type A behavior pattern. This finding suggested that Type A behavior and telic dominance might be additive or interactive in their effects on cardiovascular reactivity. Svebak, Nordby, and

Öhman (1987) tested this hypothesis in a two-factor split-plot experiment that recruited participants who were either high or low in telic dominance and in Type A behavior. Results confirmed that during perceptual-motor task performance, participants who scored high in telic dominance as well as Type A behavior pattern responded with particularly marked cardiovascular reactivity as compared with paratelic-dominant and low Type A individuals. This experiment involved no extrinsic manipulation of threat, but response magnitudes among the telic Type A participants were, nevertheless, approximately twice those of the other groups and were in the range of 30 beats per minute above resting baseline levels.

Pulse transit time was also measured in the experiment by Svebak et al. (1987). This is a noninvasive and continuous method for the measurement of systolic blood pressure changes. Svebak et al. reported patterns for systolic blood pressure changes that paralleled those for heart rate: Systolic blood pressure increases were marked among telic-dominant Type A individuals during task performance. Thus, overall, the cardiovascular findings paralleled the EMG response patterns, indicating that telic-dominant individuals (and particularly those who are also Type A) experience marked increases in cardiovascular activity during task performance, especially under conditions of threat. These findings suggest that these individuals may be at greater risk for stress-related cardiovascular illnesses.

Most of these laboratory studies recruited participants on the basis of their responses to the Telic Dominance Scale (TDS). It has been a continuous methodological challenge to assess metamotivational states in any particular situation such as in the laboratory. An extremely dominant individual may have a higher probability than one who is balanced for also being in that state in the laboratory. However, even with dominant individuals, reversal theory assumes that they reverse to the opposite mode from time to time. This may happen in the laboratory, and metamotivational state over the course of an experiment may fluctuate and may do so more with balanced than with mode-dominant individuals. Thus, Gallacher and Beswick (1988) measured blood pressure reactivity in 225 randomly recruited men exposed to four conditions (rest, mental arithmetic, reaction time, intermittent noise exposure at 90 dB). All completed the Jenkins Activity Survey for Type A behavior and a state measure to assess telic–paratelic state in the experimental situation ("How playful or serious did you feel during the experiment?"). The highest increases of systolic blood pressure occurred among the telic Type B individuals during mental arithmetic and reaction time performance, whereas the telic Type A participants responded in the moderate range. The problem of reversal in cardiovascular research has been illustrated in greater depth elsewhere in this book (see Chapter 7).

STRESSFUL LIFE EVENTS

Cortisol is secreted from the adrenal cortex as the predominant adrenocorticosteroid hormone. This major stress hormone is of vital importance for maintenance of life because of its catabolic effects on protein and glucose metabolism. However, it is also of importance to the development of immune deficiency because of its anti-inflammatory functions when tissue damage provides cortisol secretion resulting in the inhibition of histamine release from the damaged area. Histamine is needed to increase the permeability of capillaries to supply the damaged tissue with proteins and other materials for healing. Many studies have demonstrated the negative effect of cortisol on immune functions by disrupting the action of lymphocytes (e.g., Claman, 1972; see also Borysenko, 1987). Lymphocytes respond to the encounter of antigens such as bacteria and viruses by the stimulation of immunoglobulins that destroy antigens by the secretion of specialized enzymes.

Martin and his colleagues (Martin, 1985; Martin, Kuiper, Olinger, & Dobbin, 1987; Martin, Kuiper, & Olinger, 1988) reported a higher prevalence of dysphoric moods among telic-dominant individuals when exposed to stressful life events. They also observed more dysphoric moods in telic-dominant individuals when a stressful experience was ongoing than when it had been resolved. This finding suggests that telic-dominant individuals may be predisposed to perceive a stressor as a threat, whereas paratelic-dominant individuals perceive stressors as challenges with inherent potential for fun and excitement.

This hypothesis was tested by Dobbin and Martin (1988), who recruited 42 undergraduate university students (18 men, 24 women) for a study. They all completed the TDS (Murgatroyd, Rushton, Apter, & Ray, 1978). The participants were also asked to describe the most stressful event or situation that they had recently experienced in their lives and to indicate whether this event had been resolved or was still ongoing. Twenty-six of the 42 participants indicated that their most stressful recent event was still unresolved at the time of participation. The participants were therefore divided into groups with resolved versus unresolved recent stressful events. Saliva samples were obtained from all the participants on arrival in the laboratory to ascertain levels of cortisol (as a measure of stress) and IgA (see Dobbin & Martin, 1988, and Hiramatsu, 1981, for validating and methodological details). IgA is an antibody found in the secretory fluids of the human body and is an important defense against antigens in the upper respiratory and gastrointestinal tracts (Tomasi, 1976).

A weak but statistically significant negative correlation was found for the association of TDS and cortisol scores ($r = -.29$, $p < .05$) owing to somewhat lower levels of cortisol among the telic-dominant participants than among the paratelic-dominant participants. In contrast, a positive correlation of the same magnitude was found for TDS and IgA scores ($r = .31$, $p < .05$), suggesting somewhat higher levels of IgA among the telic-dominant participants than among paratelic-dominant participants.

Of particular interest in this study was the interaction between telic dominance and stress in predicting cortisol levels. As predicted, results of a hierarchical multiple regression analysis revealed a significant interaction between the TDS and the dichotomously scored resolved–unresolved stressor, indicating a

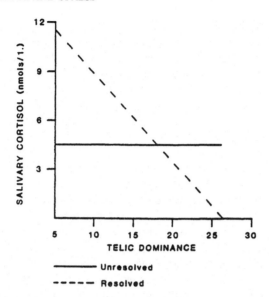

Figure 2 The relation between metamotivational dominance (continuum from telic to paratelic) and salivary cortisol for participants with resolved and unresolved recent life stressors. From "Telic Versus Paratelic Dominance: Personality Moderator of Biochemical Responses to Stress," by J. P. Dobbin & R. A. Martin, in *Progress in Reversal Theory*, edited by M. J. Apter, J. H. Kerr, and M. P. Cowles, 1988, pp. 107–116. Copyright 1988 by Elsevier. Adapted with permission.

moderation effect of telic versus paratelic dominance on the relation between stress and levels of cortisol, $F(1, 35) = 6.01$, $p < .02$. Figure 2 illustrates this interaction, showing the relation between telic dominance and salivary cortisol among the subsamples of participants with resolved versus unresolved recent stressful life events. As seen in this figure, among participants with unresolved recent stressful life events there was no association between telic dominance and cortisol secretion, whereas participants with resolved stressful life events had high levels of salivary cortisol if they were paratelic-dominant, but particularly low cortisol levels if they were telic-dominant (see dotted line in Figure 2).

This pattern of interaction indicates that telic-dominant individuals have higher cortisol levels when they are experiencing unresolved problems as compared with when their problems are resolved. In contrast, the paratelic-dominant individuals reflected a pattern for cortisol, suggesting higher levels of this stress hormone when they were relatively free of challenging problems to deal with. This interpretation is in concert with the "butterfly" illustration of relations between hedonic tone and felt arousal (given in Figure 1A, Chapter 1): High levels of felt arousal are unpleasant (anxiety) in the telic state and low levels of felt arousal are unpleasant (boredom) in the paratelic state. In both cases, dysphoria provokes elevated levels of cortisol.

These findings for cortisol were incorporated in the analysis of salivary IgA among the participants. Accordingly, IgA scores were predicted in a hierarchical regression model with all three variables (cortisol level, telic dominance, resolved–unresolved stressor) to examine a possible influence of the stress-moderating effect of telic dominance on cortisol in the secretion of IgA (see Figure 3). Results from this analysis confirmed a significant three-way interaction, $F(1, 31) = 5.98$, $p < .05$. For telic-dominant participants, IgA scores were high when cortisol scores were high, and it made little difference whether the event was resolved or not ($r = .71$, $p < .008$, and $r = .54$, $p < .05$, respectively). In contrast, for paratelic-dominant individuals, IgA and cortisol scores were positively correlated when stressful events were unresolved ($r = .17$), albeit not statistically significant, but they were negatively correlated when stressful events were resolved ($r = -.63$, $p < .05$; high cortisol levels with low IgA levels).

In summary, the findings for cortisol were generally consistent with predictions. They indicated that successful coping with stressful life events in the telic mode may provide an effect that is medically beneficial in terms of reduced cortisol secretion. This effect was also indicated among telic-dominant individuals with IgA in whom this immune function was increasingly active with higher levels of cortisol. However, a more complex mechanism seemed to be implicated for IgA among the paratelic-dominant individuals. One possible interpretation at this point is that absence of unresolved stressful events means boredom owing to lack of challenge in everyday life and that one biological correlate of boredom is a reduced secretion of IgA with increased cortisol secretion. Effortful active coping with challenges may thus provide opportunities for fun and promote immune function among paratelic-dominant individuals due to

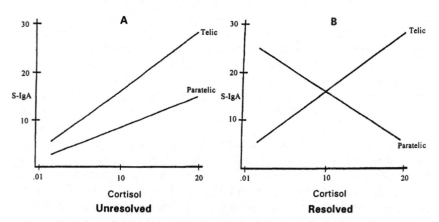

Figure 3 Relations between cortisol and salivary IgA for telic- and paratelic-dominant participants with recent life stressors that were resolved and unresolved. From "Telic Versus Paratelic Dominance: Personality Moderator of Biochemical Responses to Stress," by J. P. Dobbin & R. A. Martin, in *Progress in Reversal Theory*, edited by M. J. Apter, J. H. Kerr, and M. P. Cowles, 1988, p. 107–116. Copyright 1988 by Elsevier. Adapted with permission.

a mechanism that is obstructed in boredom. It remains a task for future research to replicate and explore this hypothesis further.

CONCLUSION

Taken together, the laboratory and field studies of responses to stressful events indicate different biological response patterns between telic- and paratelic-dominant individuals. These differences involve musculoskeletal tension patterns and cardiovascular reactivity magnitudes as well as immune-related responses to stressful life events. Among paratelic-dominant individuals, responses indicate low risk of enduring muscle tension and increased risk of acute high muscle force output as well as moderate cardiovascular activation with threat. Conversely, these individuals appear to respond with a reduction of IgA secretion with boredom (a form of tension-stress; see Chapter 2) as well as with elevated secretion of cortisol. For telic-dominant individuals, unintended muscle tension and cardiovascular response magnitudes appear to be larger with threat, and cardiovascular reactivity seems to be mediated by coronary-prone Type A behavior in threatening situations. Successful coping with everyday stressful events seems to result in low cortisol secretion, whereas IgA secretion seems to be positively associated with increased levels of cortisol secretion. Conversely, IgA deficiency appears to be associated with boredom. Taken together, these findings indicate several psychobiological relations that distinguish between telic- and paratelic-dominant individuals and make them vulnerable to different kinds of health problems under different circumstances.

REFERENCES

Apter, M. J. (1989). *Reversal theory: Motivation, emotion and personality*. London: Routledge.

Apter, M. J., & Svebak, S. (1989). Reversal theory as a biological approach to individual differences. In A. Gale & M. W. Eysenck (Eds.), *Handbook of individual differences: Biological perspectives* (pp. 323–353). Chichester, England: Wiley.

Baker, J. (1988). Stress appraisals and coping with everyday hassles. In M. J. Apter, J. H. Kerr, & M. P. Cowles (Eds.), *Progress in reversal theory* (pp. 117–128). Amsterdam: Elsevier.

Borysenko, M. (1987). The immune system: An overview. *Annals of Behavioral Medicine, 9*, 3–10.

Claman, H. N. (1972). Corticosteroids and lymphoid cells. *The New England Journal of Medicine, 24*, 388–397.

Dobbin, J. P., & Martin, R. A. (1988). Telic versus paratelic dominance: Personality moderator of biochemical responses to stress. In M. J. Apter, J. H. Kerr, & M. P. Cowles (Eds.), *Progress in reversal theory* (pp. 107–115). Amsterdam: Elsevier.

Fox, E. L. (1984). *Sports physiology*. Tokyo: Holt-Saunders International.

Gallacher, J. E. J., & Beswick, A. D. (1988). Telic state, Type A and blood pressure. In M. J. Apter, J. H. Kerr, & M. P. Cowles (Eds.), *Progress in reversal theory* (pp. 173–178). Amsterdam: Elsevier.

Hiramatsu, R. (1981). Direct assay of cortisol in human saliva by solid phase radioimmunoassay and its clinical applications. *Clinica Chimica Acta, 117*, 239–249.

Kerr, J. H., & Svebak, S. (1989). Motivational aspects of preference for, and participation in, "risk" and "safe" sports. *Personality and Individual Differences, 10,* 797–800.

Malmo, R. B. (1965). Activation: A neurophysiological dimension. *Psychological Bulletin, 64,* 225–234.

Martin, R. A. (1985). Telic dominance, stress and moods. In M. J. Apter, D. Fontana, & S. Murgatroyd (Eds.), *Reversal theory: Applications and developments* (pp. 59–71). Cardiff, Wales: University College Cardiff Press.

Martin, R. A., Kuiper, N. A., & Olinger, L. J. (1988). Telic versus paratelic dominance as a moderator of stress. In M. J. Apter, J. H. Kerr, & M. P. Cowles (Eds.), *Progress in reversal theory* (pp. 91–105). Amsterdam: Elsevier.

Martin, R. A., Kuiper, N. A., Olinger, L. J., & Dobbin, J. (1987). Is stress always bad?: Telic versus paratelic dominance as a stress-moderating variable. *Journal of Personality and Social Psychology, 53,* 970–982.

Murgatroyd, S. (1981). Reversal theory: A new perspective on crisis counseling. *British Journal of Guidance and Counseling, 9,*180–193.

Murgatroyd, S., Rushton, C., Apter, M. J., & Ray, C. (1978). The developkent of the telic dominance scale. *Journal of Personality Assessment, 42,* 519–528.

Svebak, S. (1984). Active and passive forearm flexor tension patterns in the continuous perceptual-motor task paradigm: The significance of motivation. *International Journal of Psychophysiology,2,* 167–176.

Svebak, S. (1986). Cardiac and somatic activation in the continuous perceptual-motor task: The significance of threat and serious-mindedness. *International Journal of Psychophysiology, 3,* 155–162.

Svebak, S., & Apter, M. J. (1984). Type A behavior and its relation to seriousmindedness (telic dominance). *Scandinavian Journal of Psychology, 25,* 161–167.

Svebak, S., Braathen, E. T., Sejersted, O. M., Bowim, B., Fauske, S., & Laberg, J. C. (1993). Electromyographic activation and proportion of fast versus slow twitch muscle fibers: A genetic disposition for psychogenic muscle tension. *International Journal of Psychophysiology, 15,* 43–49.

Svebak, S., & Kerr, J. (1989). The role of impulsivity in preference for sports. *Personality and Individual Differences, 10,* 51–58.

Svebak, S., & Murgatroyd, S. (1985). Metamotivational dominance: A multimethod validation of reversal theory constructs. *Personality and Social Psychology, 48,* 107–116.

Svebak, S., Nordby, H., & Öhman, A. (1987). The personality of the cardiac responder: Interaction of seriousmindedness and Type A behavior. *Biological Psychology, 25,* 1–9.

Svebak, S., Storfjell, O., & Dalen, K. (1982). The effect of a threatening context upon motivation and task-induced physiological changes. *British Journal of Psychology, 73,* 505–512.

Svebak, S., & Stoyva, J. (1980). High arousal can be pleasant and exciting: The theory of psychological arousals. *Biofeedback and Self-Regulation, 5,* 439–444.

Svebak, S., Ursin, H., Endresen, I. M., Hjelmen, A. M., & Apter, M. J. (1991). Back pain and the experience of stress, efforts and moods. *Psychology and Health, 5,* 307–314.

Tomasi, T. B. (1976). *The immune system of secretions.* Englewood Cliffs, NJ: Prentice Hall.

7

Cardiovascular Reactivity and Mode-Dominance Misfit

John Spicer and Antonia C. Lyons

Reversal theory provides a systematic approach to the study of cardiovascular reactivity, a physiological mechanism that may help explain associations between psychological attributes and processes and the risk of cardiovascular diseases such as hypertension. The authors present results from an experiment that examined the joint effects of telic–paratelic mode and dominance, arousal, and anxiety on diastolic blood pressure reactivity during conversation in 102 female students. Reactivity was highest in participants who were telic dominant but in paratelic mode and experiencing relatively high anxiety. The authors discuss the notion of mode-dominance misfit as a promising way of applying reversal theory to cardiovascular reactivity and review some of the interpretive problems encountered with this strategy.

HYPERTENSION AND CARDIOVASCULAR REACTIVITY

Hypertension continues to be a common disorder in many countries and to make a substantial contribution to morbidity and mortality from a range of consequent diseases. In New Zealand, for example, over 25% of the population aged 45 years or older are hypertensive by standard World Health Organization criteria (Nye, Paulin, & Russell, 1992). The limited success of physical aetiological explanations of hypertension has helped stimulate the search for psychological and social risk factors (Julius & Bassett, 1987). Recently, particular attention has been paid to psychological factors that appear to be related to cardiovascular reactivity. This approach suggests that the hypertension-prone person reacts to stressful situations with cardiovascular changes, notably in blood pressure, that are unusually large relative to the demands of the situation and to those exhibited by others in the same situation. Such hyperreactivity is thought to recur often over periods of years and to be sufficient to result in pathological changes in the regulation and structure of the cardiovascular system (Manuck, Kasprowicz, & Muldoon, 1990).

Recent reviews of the psychophysiological literature on cardiovascular reactivity and hypertension have reached strikingly different conclusions. For example, Carroll (1992, p. 32) claimed that "there are reasons for implicating large-magnitude, excessive cardiac reactions to stress in the development of hypertension." In contrast, Rosenman (1994, p. 38) concluded that "the findings clearly fail to support old hypotheses about causal roles of anxiety, stress and cardiovascular reactivity in the pathogenesis of sustained hypertension." These differing views turn on many complex issues, both conceptual and technical. The particular issue the present authors wish to highlight is the relative absence of psychological theory in this area and, consequently, the attractions of a reversal theory approach.

In the cardiovascular reactivity context, the fundamental task for the psychologist is to identify the psychological characteristics of the reactive individual and those of the situations in which the reactivity occurs. Evidence to date has suggested that blood pressure reactivity may be notable in individuals who are chronically hostile (Suls & Wan, 1993), exhibit Type A behavior (Van Egeren & Sparrow, 1990), and have low social support (Kamarck, Manuck, & Jennings, 1990) and also in situations involving active coping with challenge (Hodapp, Bongard, & Heiligtag, 1992) and conversation (Naring, de Mey, & Schaap, 1988), especially with strangers (Spitzer, Llabre, Ironson, Gellman, & Schneiderman, 1992).

. There are various points to note about this list of characteristics. First, the total database is still small and often internally inconsistent, so the list is far from definitive. Second, the characteristics represent a wide range of construct types. Third, many of the contributing studies have analyzed one characteristic at a time, providing at best a piecemeal account of complex psychological processes. Fourth, and most germane to this discussion, the characteristics are rarely found in developed psychological theory. This has become particularly apparent as researchers begin to study combinations of characteristics and find, for example, that hostility and reactivity are linked most clearly in relevant social settings such as harassment and arguments (Smith & Christensen, 1992). There is a strong need for psychological theory to guide reactivity research and to help interpret the findings. In practice, interpretations tend to be rather post hoc, to be based on common sense, and to be limited in scope. The present authors believe that reversal theory has considerable potential in this context, as they hope to demonstrate in this chapter.

REVERSAL THEORY AND CARDIOVASCULAR REACTIVITY

Reversal theory has various general features that suggest its potential utility in research on reactivity and cardiovascular diseases such as hypertension. It constitutes a framework within which a wide range of psychological constructs—

notably motives, emotions, and personality attributes—may be integrated. Further, its particular emphasis on psychological states, such as arousal and meta-motivational modes, provides a strong platform from which to view the details of the actual psychophysiological interface. The theory can also be applied to the dual time frames of the reactivity-disease hypothesis: the transient reactive episode and the long-term accumulation of risk, perhaps by means of distinctive patterning of reversals and the notion of mode dominance. Finally, because reversal theory has already been used as a basis for developing interventions in a number of areas such as mental health, any aetiological explanations it provides for physical diseases, such as hypertension, could be systematically linked to subsequent preventive strategies.

Attempts have been made to apply reversal theory to aspects of cardiovascular reactivity. These include theoretical reinterpretations of Type A behavior (Svebak, 1988) and empirical research that combines Type A behavior with reversal theory constructs (Svebak, Nordby, & Öhman, 1987). The empirical attempts to study the joint effects of Type A behavior and reversal theory constructs on blood pressure have met with mixed success (Gallacher & Beswick, 1988). Given the many theoretical and methodological problems that continue to beset the Type A pattern, the present authors have doubts about the wisdom of pursuing this line of integrative research, at least until Svebak's (1988) reinterpretations have been developed further. His basic argument was that Type A coronary-prone behavior equals the constellation of telic dominance (relating to unpleasant feelings of high arousal, especially in the form of anger), mastery dominance (corresponding to Type A competitiveness and the need to control), negativistic dominance (corresponding to Type A hostility), and autic dominance.

Psychophysiological work that has focused solely on reversal theory constructs (e.g., Svebak, 1986) has produced generally encouraging results, as Apter (1989) concluded in his extensive review. For the present purposes, the most notable emergent theme from this research concerns telic–paratelic mode and dominance. Results from various studies have suggested that higher cardiovascular reactivity, especially heart rate, is exhibited by people who are telic-dominant or in telic mode. In the experiment described below the present authors pursued this theme, but tried to do so in ways that avoided certain limitations of work to date.

Although one of the strengths of reversal theory is that it differentiates a great variety of psychological states in a very systematic way, the design of many of the psychophysiological studies has made it very difficult, and sometimes impossible, to detect differential effects. Thus, it is often difficult to decide whether physiological effects are due to mode, dominance, or states such as arousal or emotions or to particular combinations of these. In the following experiment, the authors tried to enable variation in telic–paratelic mode and dominance, arousal level, and anxiety and to measure their separate and joint effects on blood pressure reactivity.

A further striking feature of psychophysiological research guided by reversal theory is the widespread use of artificial stressors, such as mental arithmetic tasks and computer games, to induce reactivity. There are strong arguments for adopting such standardized strategies but when subsequent attempts are made to link reactivity to disease, the problem of ecological validity arises. In this chronic-disease context it is important to demonstrate not only that certain processes are possible, but also that they are likely to occur with reasonable frequency and consistency in everyday life. Accordingly, the authors decided to use self-focused conversation as the stressor in the following experiment. In addition to concerns about ecological validity, this choice was also guided by evidence that shows that conversation is a particularly reliable inducer of reactivity (Lassner, Matthews, & Stoney, 1994) and by Fontana's (1988) hypotheses on the link between the telic state and self-awareness.

The final noteworthy feature is the issue of gender differences. As has been discussed elsewhere (Spicer & Chamberlain, 1996), women continue to be under-studied in cardiovascular research, despite their proneness to cardiovascular disease and despite demonstrated gender differences in reactivity (Girdler, Turner, Sherwood, & Light, 1990) and in relevant psychological attributes (Linden, Chambers, Maurice, & Lenz, 1993). Even where women are included as participants, their results are often merged with those of men or no attempts are made to test formally for gender-related interactions. From the reversal theory perspective, it appears that the issue of gender differences has received little attention. These concerns led the present authors to study only female participants in the following experiment.

In summary, the authors believe that reversal theory has considerable potential for analyses of the psychophysiology of cardiovascular reactivity, which subsequently might contribute to aetiological explanations of cardiovascular diseases such as hypertension. The remainder of this chapter describes an experiment in which the authors tested whether the blood pressure reactivity of women engaged in self-related conversation was associated with telic–paratelic mode and dominance, anxiety state, and arousal state, singly or in combination. Reversal theory seemed to suggest particular sensitivity to the combined effects of these variables, as theoretically they jointly capture more differentiated states. So the authors were especially interested in the possibility of detecting interaction effects, though they had no strong expectations as to their precise form.

EXPERIMENTAL METHOD

The experiment was completed by 102 female student volunteers aged between 18–43 years ($M = 21.4$, $SD = 4.7$). All experimental sessions were conducted by Antonia C. Lyons in a standard laboratory setting. Each student was engaged in conversation for 3–6 min about some aspect of herself that she had chosen from a list consisting of options such as "my personal goals" or "habits I would like to change." The participant's systolic and diastolic blood pressure and heart rate were taken every minute during a prior 4-min rest period spent relaxing, then during at least 3 min of talk, using an automated device, the Critikon Dinamap 8100. These measurement and recording operations were computer controlled, and results were accumulated in a computer file for later analysis. The primary dependent variable, blood pressure reactivity, was defined as average change in blood pressure from baseline to conversation, where baseline was defined as the second half of the rest period (Llabre, Spitzer, Saab, Ironson, & Schneiderman, 1991).

Immediately after the conversation, participants rated the telic–paratelic mode and the arousal level they had experienced during the conversation, using the 6-point serious–playful and low–high arousal items from the Telic State Measure (Svebak, Storfjell, & Dalen, 1982). Scores were dichotomized (1–3 and 4–6) for the analyses below, following earlier practice. Participants also rated the anxiety level they had experienced during the conversation using the bipolar form of the Profile of Mood States (POMS-BI; Educational and Industrial Testing Service, 1982). This well-established measure contains six *anxious* items (tense, nervous, jittery, shaky, anxious, uneasy) and six *composed* items (composed, untroubled, peaceful, serene, calm, relaxed), each of which individuals rated on a 4-point scale. Their POMS score was the sum of their composed ratings, minus the sum of their anxiety ratings, plus a constant of 18 to avoid negative scores. Finally, participants completed the Telic Dominance Scale (Murgatroyd, Rushton, Apter, & Ray, 1978), and their seriousness subscale score was used as an indicator of dominance, again following earlier practice of other researchers.

RESULTS AND DBP REACTIVITY

Although reactivity was measured as changes in systolic and diastolic blood pressure (DBP) and in heart rate, virtually all of the statistically significant effects occurred with respect to DBP. Accordingly, the results and discussion focus on DBP reactivity. Overall, the talking condition produced a significant DBP increase from baseline of about 10 mmHg on average. This fits reassuringly with earlier findings on how conversation affects blood pressure and shows that the particular technique used in this study was effective in evoking reactivity.

The main and interactive effects of dominance, mode, anxiety and arousal on DBP change were tested by using analysis of covariance (ANCOVA) programs of SPSS/PC+. Mode and arousal were treated as dichotomous factors, and dominance and anxiety were entered as continuous covariates. Because the design was unbalanced, a regression approach was used that controlled for all same and lower order effects. It is also worth noting that only two of the independent variables were significantly correlated: Arousal was correlated .34 with anxiety. This reassures about confounding of the variables included and also suggests that the theoretical constructs were empirically well separated.

The ANCOVA produced a significant main effect for telic dominance, $F(1, 81) = 5.83$, $p < .05$, which showed that telic-dominant women displayed greater DBP increases on average than paratelic-dominant women. However, the presence of several significant interaction effects suggested that the picture is more complex than this. There were two-way interaction effects for Dominance × Mode, $F(1, 81) = 8.11$, $p < .01$; Dominance × Anxiety, $F(1, 81) = 4.13$, $p < .05$; and Anxiety × Arousal, $F(1, 81) = 4.04$, $p < .05$, and a three-way interaction for Dominance × Mode × Anxiety, $F(1, 81) = 3.89$, $p < .05$. All other effects were clearly nonsignificant, using a two-tailed alpha of .05. To explore the interaction effects, the dominance and anxiety variables were dichotomized at their medians and mean DBP change scores were plotted for all relevant subgroups. (To keep this account focused and relatively brief, the Anxiety × Arousal effect is not referred to further. Further details are available from the authors.)

The shape of the Dominance × Mode interaction is shown in Figure 1. Overall, women who were telic-dominant exhibited greater DBP change, as the main effect indicated. However, the effect was much more marked for telic-dominant women who were in paratelic mode: that is, those who generally preferred to be serious but who felt playful when talking about themselves. This is the seriously playful misfit to which the title of this chapter alludes. In addition to the distinctive misfit nature of this effect, the size of the blood pressure increase, which approached 15 mmHg in this subgroup, is also striking.

Taking anxiety into account produced an even more striking three-way effect, shown in Figure 2. The subgroup showing the greatest DBP change by a considerable margin was that of the telic-dominant women, who were in paratelic

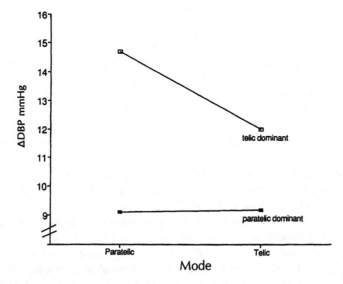

Figure 1   The effects of dominance and mode on change in diastolic blood pressure (DBP).

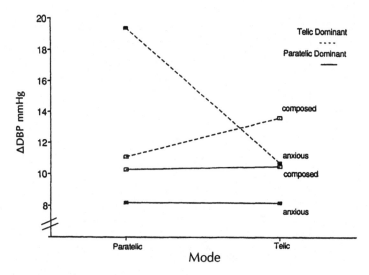

Figure 2 The effects of dominance, mode, and anxiety on change in diastolic blood pressure (DBP).

mode but who were also experiencing anxiety. As the figure shows, the average DBP increase in this subgroup was nearly 20 mmHg. It is important to emphasize that this pattern does not represent a sequence of events. A misfit of dominance and mode was not found to be associated with greater anxiety. So the striking DBP increase was present only in the subgroup of misfits who reported anxiety.

Anxiety also interacted with dominance in a way that suggests another type of misfit effect, as shown in Figure 3. This pattern draws attention to the reactivity of paratelic-dominant women who did not feel anxious, that is, they were relatively composed, given the bipolar nature of the POMS-BI measure. The shape of the interaction suggests that, among the paratelic-dominant women, those who were composed showed greater DBP change than those who were anxious. This is consistent with the notion that paratelic individuals may find being relaxed a stressful state, as they tend to seek the feeling of arousal. This interpretation is very speculative and is not consistent with all of the data. Nevertheless, the pattern does encourage one to look at the paratelic- as well as the telic-dominant group and to think about possible misfits in more than one way.

DISCUSSION OF THE FINDINGS

These results give added weight to the contention that reversal theory provides a potentially fruitful approach to the psychophysiology of cardiovascular reactivity. The pattern of results has several interesting features. The absence of main effects, other than for telic dominance, supports the notion that the physiological substrate of reversal states, modes, and dominance is more likely to be

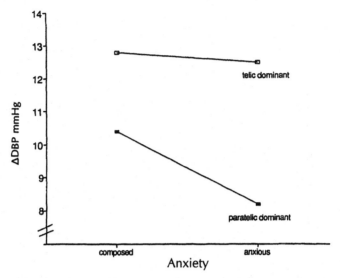

Figure 3 The effects of dominance and anxiety on change in diastolic blood pressure (DBP).

discernible when the psychological differentiation provided by the theory is exploited. Thus, these data show no independent effects of arousal, anxiety, or telic mode on DBP reactivity, but all emerge as influential in some way when their interactions are considered. Moreover, the strength of the effects is far from negligible, and certainly is of clinical interest. Similarly, the restriction of the effects to DBP reactivity (other than a main effect of telic dominance on systolic blood pressure reactivity) does not diminish their clinical relevance. Although the evidence is mixed (Pickering & Gerin, 1992), there is some indication that DBP reactivity is one of the best single cardiovascular predictors of subsequent hypertension (Chaney & Eyman, 1988, cited in Pickering & Gerin, 1992).

The most interesting feature of the results is the appearance of what the authors have termed misfit effects, especially that between paratelic mode and telic dominance. It is particularly striking that this effect appears to be asymmetric. In the present sample, women who were paratelic dominant did not exhibit enhanced reactivity when in telic mode. Thus, it seems that only certain types of misfit may have physiological consequences.

The notion that forms of psychological or social misfit may be pathogenic has previously emerged in health psychology in various ways. For example, complex theories have been elaborated by Moss (1973) on biosocial resonation and by Totman (1979) on the failure to register consistency between actions and social rules. More recently and specifically, Engebretson, Matthews, and Scheier (1989) have reported an intriguing misfit effect for anger and blood pressure reactivity. They found that reactivity was higher in participants who typically preferred to suppress anger but were induced to express it in an experimental task, and in those with the opposite pattern, than in participants for whom the preference and induced expression matched. Similarly, the present authors have recently reported an association between cynical hostility and resting blood pressure, specific to women, which they have interpreted as symptomatic of a mismatch between attitudes and gender-specific social rules (Spicer & Chamberlain, 1996).

It is suggested that interaction, and particularly mode-dominance misfit, effects are a promising avenue for exploration in psychophysiological research on reversal theory. However, this approach highlights various problems needing attention, some of which arise in the present study and others of which relate to reversal theory in general. The central problem highlighted by the present study concerns the three-way interaction that shows that reactivity was highest in women who were telic-dominant and reported being in paratelic mode and feeling anxious during conversation. The problem here is that, according to reversal theory, people in paratelic mode should not experience anxiety, because any high arousal is felt as excitement or as some other form of pleasant high-arousal emotion. It is possible that the mode measurement—a single, dichotomized rating scale completed retrospectively—was inadequate. Perhaps not all of this subgroup were actually in paratelic mode during the conversation, especially given their telic dominance. However, this mode assessment was similar to that used in other studies, and in other respects it produced coherent results. Whatever the resolution of this particular puzzle, it is clear that developing effective measures of reversal theory states is still a need that has only been partially met (Cook, Gerkovich, Potocky, & O'Connell, 1993).

Naturally it is preferable to suspect that the present problem lies more with the assessment of anxiety. The most obvious suggestion here would be that the POMS-BI scores in this subgroup might have been relatively high, but not high enough to indicate anxiety as such. This interpretation is particularly attractive given the bipolar nature and scoring system of the measure described in the Experiment Method section above. However, inspection of the scores in this subgroup revealed that they fell high in the normative range provided in the POMS-BI manual. If the POMS-BI successfully measures anxiety, then these participants were clearly reporting high levels of anxiety.

This statement, in turn, raises the question of whether the POMS-BI scores actually captured some other state such as arousal or hedonic tone, which would be compatible with the paratelic mode. The former suggestion lacks force because arousal was measured in its own right, and, although it proved to be correlated with anxiety, this relationship was statistically controlled in the analyses. So any anxiety effects on DBP reactivity are net of those due to arousal. The hedonic tone interpretation is more plausible, especially as Martin (1985) has used the total POMS-BI score across all subscales as an indicator of this construct and found associations between stress effects and telic dominance that were strikingly in accord with reversal theory predictions.

An alternative interpretation, even more in keeping with reversal theory propositions, is that those participants reporting anxiety in the paratelic state were in fact experiencing parapathic anxiety (see Chapter 2). Parapathic anxiety has the same "feeling" as its normal counterpart but is placed in an interpretive frame that protects the individual from its usual significance (Apter, 1989, pp. 43–46). An example would be the anxiety experienced during a suspenseful movie, where the entertainment context places the viewer in a "safety zone" frame. A key feature of parapathic emotions is that, according to reversal theory, they can only be experienced in paratelic mode. Participants in this experiment may have felt threatened by the requirement to talk about themselves and by the physiological monitoring equipment. However, the encouragement to relax, the friendly manner of the experimenter, the explicit reassurances about confidentiality, and the implied safety of a university laboratory could have provided participants with a paratelic safety zone within which their anxiety would be interpreted.

The general problem remains, though, of interpreting findings from studies that combine constructs and measures from within and without reversal theory. This point was touched on earlier with respect to Type A behavior, but the anxiety example provides a more compelling illustration of the problem. The POMS-BI Anxious–Composed subscale provides a reliable and valid measure of what is usually understood as anxiety, successfully differentiating it from a variety of other emotional states. However, by its very nature it, or any other anxiety scale, does not provide the opportunity for a respondent who is feeling aroused to report this as excitement or as parapathic anxiety, key alternative interpretations in reversal theory terms. When results not congruent with reversal theory are obtained, which is deficient: the theory, the construct, or the measure, and how can one tell? A purist line would presumably suggest that this dilemma should be avoided by developing all constructs and measures from the ground up inside reversal theory and avoiding studies that use imported constructs and measures, unless they happen to fit the theory's constraints. Given the range of the theory, however, this would involve a paralyzing burden of reconceptualization and psychometric development in the area of the emotions alone, not to mention the potential marginalization of many of the useful products of psychological enquiry. There are no ready answers to this dilemma, but it is suggested that it is fundamental to the development and wider acceptance of reversal theory.

The use of a social stimulus, while appropriate for the reasons given earlier, also raises concerns similar to those voiced in the preceding paragraph. Although the constructs of mode, dominance, arousal, and anxiety were taken from within the confines of reversal theory, this was not the case for the social stimulus of a personal conversation. Progress has been made in developing reversal theory accounts of social stressors (e.g., Svebak, 1991), but these did not appear to fit the needs of this experiment. Given the emerging importance of social stressors in the evocation of cardiovascular reactivity, further theorization

of the social environment would seem to be a high priority for psychophysiological research in reversal theory.

CONCLUSION

As the findings are interpreted, they clearly require replication in women and
men before being accorded too much weight. More generally, it would be advis-
able to extend the psychophysiological research focus beyond the telic–paratelic
modes, however beguiling the results, and to pay considerably more attention to
the transactional modes (mastery–sympathy and alloic–autic). The notion of mode-
dominance misfit was discussed as a promising way of applying reversal theory.
Now it seems that trying to pinpoint reversal theory states more firmly in the
social environment would be a worthwhile objective for future research in this
area.

REFERENCES

Apter, M. J. (1989). *Reversal theory: Motivation, emotion and personality*. London: Rout-
ledge.
Carroll, D. (1992). *Health psychology: Stress, behavior and disease*. London: Falmer Press.
Cook, M. R., Gerkovich, M. M., Potocky, M., & O'Connell, K. A. (1993). Instruments for the
assessment of reversal theory states. *Patient Education and Counseling, 22*, 99–106.
Educational and Industrial Testing Service. (1982). Profile of mood states: Bi-polar form (POMS-
BI). San Diego, CA: Author.
Engebretson, T. O., Matthews, K. A., & Scheier, M. F. (1989). Relations between anger expres-
sion and cardiovascular reactivity: Reconciling inconsistent findings through a matching
hypothesis. *Journal of Personality and Social Psychology, 57*, 513–521.
Fontana, D. (1988). Self-awareness and self-forgetting: Now I see me, now I don't. In M. J.
Apter, J. H. Kerr, & M. P. Cowles (Eds.), *Progress in reversal theory* (pp. 349–357).
Amsterdam: Elsevier.
Gallacher, J. E. J., & Beswick, A. D. (1988). Telic state, Type A and blood pressure. In M. J.
Apter, J. H. Kerr, & M. P. Cowles (Eds.), *Progress in reversal theory* (pp. 173–178).
Amsterdam: Elsevier.
Girdler, S. S., Turner, J. R., Sherwood, A., & Light, K. C. (1990). Gender differences in blood
pressure control during a variety of behavioral stressors. *Psychosomatic Medicine, 52*, 571–
591.
Hodapp, V., Bongard, S., & Heiligtag, U. (1992). Active coping, expression of anger and cardio-
vascular reactivity. *Personality and Individual Differences, 13*, 1069–1076.
Julius, S., & Bassett, D. R. (Eds.). (1987). *Behavioral factors in hypertension*. Amsterdam: Elsevier.
Kamarck, T. W., Manuck, S. B., & Jennings, J. R. (1990). Social support reduces cardiovascular
reactivity to psychological challenge: A laboratory model. *Psychosomatic Medicine, 52*, 42–
58.
Lassner, J. B., Matthews, K. A., & Stoney, C. M. (1994). Are cardiovascular reactors to asocial
stress also reactors to social stress? *Journal of Personality and Social Psychology, 66*, 69–
77.
Linden, W., Chambers, L., Maurice, J., & Lenz, J. W. (1993). Sex differences in social support,
self-deception, hostility and ambulatory cardiovascular activity. *Health Psychology, 12*, 376–
380.
Llabre, M. M., Spitzer, S. B., Saab, P. G., Ironson, G. H., & Schneiderman, N. (1991). The

reliability and specificity of delta versus residualized change as measures of cardiovascular reactivity to behavioral challenges. *Psychophysiology, 28,* 701–711.

Manuck, S. B., Kasprowicz, A. L., & Muldoon, M. F. (1990). Behaviorally evoked cardiovascular reactivity and hypertension: Conceptual issues and potential associations. *Annals of Behavioral Medicine, 12,* 17–29.

Martin, R. (1985). Telic dominance, stress and moods. In M. J. Apter, D. Fontana, & S. Murgatroyd (Eds.), *Reversal theory: Applications and developments* (pp. 59–71). Cardiff, Wales: University College Cardiff Press.

Moss, G. E. (1973). *Illness, immunity and social interaction: The dynamics of biosocial resonation.* New York: Wiley.

Murgatroyd, S., Rushton, C., Apter, M., & Ray, C. (1978). The development of the Telic Dominance Scale. *Journal of Personality Assessment, 42,* 519–528.

Naring, G. W., de Mey, H. R., & Schaap, C. P. (1988). Blood pressure response during verbal interaction: Review and prospect. *Current Psychological Research and Reviews, 7,* 187–198.

Nye, E. R., Paulin, J., & Russell, D. G. (1992). Blood pressure in a random sample of the New Zealand population. *The New Zealand Medical Journal, 105,* 1–3.

Pickering, T. G., & Gerin, W. (1992). Does cardiovascular reactivity have pathogenic significance in hypertensive patients? In E. H. Johnson, W. D. Gentry, & S. Julius, *Personality, elevated blood pressure and essential hypertension* (pp. 151–173). Washington: Hemisphere.

Rosenman, R. H. (1994). Some effects of the environment on emotions and their relationships to cardiovascular diseases. In J. Rose (Ed.), *Human stress and the environment* (pp. 27–58). Yverdon, Switzerland: Gorden & Breach.

Smith, T. W., & Christensen, A. J. (1992). Cardiovascular reactivity and interpersonal relations: Psychosomatic processes in social context. *Journal of Social and Clinical Psychology, 11,* 279–301.

Spicer, J., & Chamberlain, K. (1996). Cynical hostility, anger and resting blood pressure. *Journal of Psychosomatic Research, 40,* 359–368.

Spitzer, S. B., Llabre, M. M., Ironson, G. H., Gellman, M. D., & Schneiderman, N. (1992). The influence of social situations on ambulatory blood pressure. *Psychosomatic Medicine, 54,* 79–86

Suls, J., & Wan, C. K. (1993). The relationship between trait hostility and cardiovascular reactivity: A quantitative review and analysis. *Psychophysiology, 30,* 615–626.

Svebak, S. (1986). Cardiac and somatic activation in the continuous perceptual-motor task: The significance of threat and serious-mindedness. *International Journal of Psychophysiology, 3,* 155–162.

Svebak, S. (1988). Personality, stress and cardiovascular risk. In M. J. Apter, J. H. Kerr, & M. P. Cowles (Eds.), *Progress in reversal theory* (pp. 163–172). Amsterdam: Elsevier.

Svebak, S. (1991). The role of effort in stress and emotion. In C. D. Spielberger, I. G. Sarason, Z. Kulcsar, & G. L. Van Heck (Eds.), *Stress and emotion* (Vol. 14, pp. 121–134). New York: Hemisphere.

Svebak, S., Nordby, H., & Öhman, A. (1987). The personality of the cardiac responder: Interaction of seriousmindedness and Type A behavior. *Biological Psychology, 25,* 1–9.

Svebak, S., Storfjell, O., & Dalen, K. (1982). The effect of a threatening context upon motivation and task-induced physiological changes. *British Journal of Psychology, 73,* 505–512.

Totman, R. (1979). *Social causes of illness.* London: Souvenir Press.

Van Egeren, L. F., & Sparrow, A. W. (1990). Ambulatory monitoring to assess real-life cardiovascular reactivity in Type A and Type B subjects. *Psychosomatic Medicine, 52,* 297–306.

III

---

*PSYCHOLOGY
AND PHYSIOLOGY
OF SMOKING*

8

Relapse Crises
During Smoking Cessation

Kathleen A. O'Connell, Mary M. Gerkovich, and Mary R. Cook

This chapter addresses the relationship of reversal theory states to lapses during smoking cessation. Descriptions of highly tempting episodes given by 56 participants who were attempting to quit smoking were coded for all four pairs of reversal theory states: telic–paratelic, negativistic–conformist, mastery–sympathy, and autic–alloic. In addition, the episodes were coded for the two versions of the autic state, intra-autic and autocentric, and for the two versions of the alloic state, allocentric and proautic. Using logit modeling, it was determined that the combination of three metamotivational state pairs (telic–paratelic, negativistic–conformist, mastery–sympathy) and the versions of the autic state provided an adequate fit to the data that included lapse–abstain as the dependent variable. The combination of the telic–paratelic pair and the interaction of the mastery–sympathy pair with intra-autic–autocentric versions of the autic state provided the best model. This study provides one of the first published reports in which all four pairs of reversal theory's metamotivational states were applied to the same data set. The findings indicate that the four pairs of states provide nonoverlapping information and illustrate the usefulness of reversal theory in identifying variables that are relevant to resisting the urge to smoke.

Cigarette smoking is a serious risk to health. Most smokers know of the dangers of smoking, and many attempt to stop. However, relapse rates are high, with 65% to 70% of those attempting to quit relapsing within 12 months of cessation (Shiffman, 1993). Moreover, there is evidence that a single lapse during a cessation attempt has a 90% probability of leading to a full-blown relapse (Brandon, Tiffany, & Baker, 1986). Because relapse is such a common outcome of cessation attempts and because an initial lapse is so dangerous, several groups of investigators have studied the relapse crises experienced by those who are trying to quit smoking (Baer, Kamarck, Lichtenstein, & Ranson, 1989; Bliss, Garvey, Heinold, & Hitchcock, 1989; O'Connell & Martin, 1987; Shiffman, 1986). A relapse crisis is defined as a situation experienced during a cessation attempt in which the individual either smokes a cigarette or is highly tempted to smoke but resists. Learning about the immediate precipitants of lapses and the concomitants of resisting the urge to smoke can yield information that promotes successful smoking cessation.

In several studies, the authors have shown that reversal theory states are useful in explaining the outcome of relapse crises. O'Connell, Cook, Gerkovich, Potocky, and Swan (1990) showed that the telic–paratelic and negativistic–conformist pairs of states were significantly related to the outcomes of the relapse crises of those who had remained abstinent or abstinent with an occasional slip for at least 3 months. The results indicated that ex-smokers in negativistic or paratelic states were significantly more likely to lapse during relapse crises than ex-smokers in telic and conformist states. These results were found both for data collected at 3 months after cessation and for data collected at later follow-ups (6 to 15 months after cessation). A subsequent study (Potocky, Gerkovich, O'Connell & Cook, 1991) replicated these results, using a within-subjects analysis. This study compared lapse and resist episodes of the same participants and showed that lapses were related to paratelic or negativistic states and resisting was associated with telic and conformist states. This study demonstrated that lapsing was associated with metamotivational state and not some enduring characteristic of the participant.

In a third study, Cook, Gerkovich, O'Connell, and Potocky (1995) investigated the relapse crises that occurred during the first 6 weeks of cessation in a new group of participants. In this data set, Cook et al. found that although the negativistic–conformist pair was unrelated to the outcome of the relapse crisis, participants in the paratelic state were significantly more likely to lapse than participants in the telic state. Using the same data set, O'Connell, Gerkovich, and Cook (1995) undertook a separate analysis of the relationships of the mastery–sympathy pair to the outcome of relapse crises. Applying a newly developed coding schedule, they found that participants in the sympathy state were significantly more likely to lapse during relapse crises than participants in the mastery state.

Each of the studies described above tested statistical models that included the reversal theory pairs and cigarette availability, a dichotomous variable indicating whether the participant had to exert effort to get a cigarette in the situations. In two of the three reports, cigarette availability was an important component of the models (Cook et al., 1995; O'Connell et al., 1995). As would be expected, when cigarettes are available with no effort, ex-smokers are more likely to lapse than when effort must be expended to get cigarettes. In one of the studies (O'Connell et al., 1990), this effect was true only in the paratelic state. Models that included both cigarette availability and reversal theory constructs as main effects correctly classified 86% to 89% of the participants as abstainers or lapsers. When cigarette availability was not accounted for in the models, single reversal theory variables correctly classified 68% to 70% of the participants as abstainers or lapsers. Previous work did not include a test of the combination of all four pairs of metamotivational states as predictors of smoking outcome. Most of the empirical work in reversal theory has focused on the telic–paratelic pair of metamotivational states. A few studies of other pairs have also been reported, but this study is one of the few that has examined the combined effect of all the metamotivational pairs in relation to a given outcome.

The purpose of the study reported in this chapter is to investigate the adequacy of a model that includes all four pairs of metamotivational states to explain smoking outcome during relapse crises. Four research questions are addressed: (a) Are the four pairs of states orthogonal to each other as Apter has posited (e.g., Apter, 1989)? (b) Does the combination of the four states provide an adequate model to account for smoking or abstaining during relapse crises? (c) Which pairs are most important in predicting smoking or abstaining during relapse crises? and (d) What percentage of the participants are correctly classified using all the states?

METHOD OF EXPLORING THE MODEL

Participants

A sample of 68 individuals who were attending community smoking cessation programs in a large city in the midwestern United States were recruited for the study. The mean age of the sample was 43 years, and 66% of the sample were women. Participants in the sample had smoked an average of 30 cigarettes a day for an average of 25 years. Participants in the study had an average of four prior quit attempts. All participants had been abstinent, except for isolated lapses, for at least 1 week after cessation.

Procedures

The Metamotivational State Interview (O'Connell, Potocky, Cook, & Gerkovich, 1991), a semistructured interview developed to assess reversal theory constructs during highly tempting situations, was used. Participants were asked about the previous 2 weeks. They described in their own words the circumstances, moods, and environments of both a lapse episode (if they had experienced one) and a highly tempting episode that was resisted. Then participants were asked specific questions about the feelings and thoughts they had at three points in time: just before the temptation, at the peak of the temptation, and at the resolution of the temptation (the point at which the participant decided whether to smoke). Codes given to the resolution coding unit were the focus of the data analysis. At each interview session, participants answered questions about their smoking behavior and provided breath samples for carbon monoxide analysis to verify their self-reported smoking status.

The Metamotivational State Coding Schedule (O'Connell et al., 1991) was used to code the data. For each of the three time points in the relapse crisis, coders determined whether the participant was telic or paratelic, negativistic or conformist, in the mastery or sympathy state, and in the autic or alloic state. In addition, coders determined which version of the autic (autocentric or intra-autic) or alloic state (allocentric or pro-autic) was operative. For each pair, a "can't-code" category was used when insufficient information was available for that particular pair. Too few instances of the alloic state were identified in the data set to warrant further analysis of the autic–alloic pair. However, each version of the autic state did occur with enough frequency to be included in the data analysis. All data were coded by two coders, and interrater reliability was 88% for both telic–paratelic and negativistic–conformist pairs and 74% for the mastery–sympathy pair. All interrater reliability coefficients were significant by the kappa statistic (Cohen, 1960). Disagreements were resolved by discussion between the coders or by a third coder. Subsequent to the determination of interrater reliability estimates, 3 of the participants were dropped from the analysis because coders determined these participants did not report the selected episode in enough detail to enable the coders to assign any of the metamotivational codes. Nine additional participants were dropped from the analysis because coders determined that the mastery–sympathy codes could not be assigned on the basis of information given.

Data Analyses

For data analysis, one relapse crisis reported during the first 6 weeks of smoking cessation was chosen for each participant. For participants who had lapsed, the first reported lapse episode was chosen. For participants who had not lapsed, the most highly tempting episode, as measured by the participants' rating of the episode on a 10-point scale, was chosen. Data were submitted to logit modeling. This is a type of categorical data analysis that allows testing of various prediction models by determining whether any significant amount of residual variance remains after a model is fit. The three pairs of states and the versions of the autic mode were used as predictor variables, and smoking status during the relapse crisis was used as the outcome variable.

WHAT THE MODEL DETERMINED

Data analyses indicated that 39% of the episodes used in the analyses were lapse episodes and 61% were abstinent episodes. In the selected episodes, 79% of the participants were telic and 21% were paratelic; 80% were conformist and 20% were negativistic; 70% were in the mastery state and 30% were in the sympathy state; 100% were in the autic state and 0% in the alloic state; and 73% were in the intra-autic version of the autic state and 27% were in the autocentric version of the autic state.

To address the first research question, which concerned whether the four pairs of states are orthogonal to each other, the associations table generated during the logit modeling procedures was examined. The associations represent the chi-square tests of the two-way associations of all the variables in the analyses. Results indicated that telic–paratelic, negativistic–conformist, and mastery–sympathy pairs were not significantly related to each other. However, the version of the autic state the participant was in was significantly related to two of the pairs. Telic participants were significantly more likely to be in the intra-autic state than were paratelic participants ($p < .05$). Conformist participants were significantly more likely to be in the intra-autic state than were negativistic participants ($p < .05$).

To address the second research question, which concerned whether the combination of the four states provides an adequate model to account for the outcome of relapse crises, a logit model was tested with the three pairs of metamotivational states and the two versions of the autic state as predictor variables and smoking outcome as the dependent variable. Because no participants were in the alloic state, the autic–alloic pair was dropped from the analyses. The preliminary associations analysis indicated that the negativistic–conformist pair was unrelated to smoking outcome. Therefore, the negativistic–conformist pair was dropped from further model testing. The associations analysis also indicated that four terms were related to smoking outcome: the telic–paratelic pair, the mastery–sympathy pair, the intra-autic–autocentric versions of the autic state, and the interaction of mastery–sympathy with intra-autic–autocentric. The combination of these four terms provided an adequate fit to the data that included smoking outcome as the dependent variable ($G^2 = 2.1$, $p = .553$).

The third research question concerned which states were most important in explaining lapses during relapse crises. This question was addressed by testing several alternative models, each of which excluded one of the predictor variables in the model. Testing of alternative models indicated that the combination of the telic–paratelic pair and the interaction of mastery–sympathy with intra-autic–autocentric versions of the autic state provided the most parsimonious model. ($G^2 = 3.9$, $p = .561$.)

The fourth research question, which addressed the percentage of participants correctly classified by the model, was addressed by computing the percentage of participants who were correctly classified as abstainers or lapsers, using the model parameters. Basically, 31 of 44 persons in the telic state were correctly classified as abstainers, and 9 of the 12 persons in the paratelic state were correctly classified as lapsers. Overall, 71% of the participants were correctly classified by using the telic–paratelic pair by itself (Table 1).

It was found through the interaction between mastery–sympathy and intra-autic–autocentric that the two state combinations are related to lapsing during the episode (Table 2). Eight of the 11 participants in the intra-autic sympathy state lapsed. Thus, 73% of the participants who were oriented toward self-care and self-indulgence during the episode succumbed to the urge to smoke. In

Table 1   Frequencies of Participants in Telic
Versus Paratelic States by Lapse Versus Abstain

Smoking outcome	Telic	Paratelic
Lapse	13	9[a]
Abstain	31[a]	3

[a]Correct predictions: 40 of 56 (71%).

addition, 6 of the 9 individuals in the autocentric mastery state lapsed, indicating that two thirds of the individuals who were oriented toward controlling others smoked during the episode. Conversely, 25 of the 30 individuals in the intra-autic mastery state abstained. Thus, 83% of those who were oriented to self-discipline resisted the urge to smoke. Overall, the interaction of mastery–sympathy with the intra-autic and autocentric versions of the autic state correctly classified 70% of the participants as smokers or abstainers.

Combining the telic–paratelic variable with the interaction of mastery–sympathy and intra-autic–autocentric states yielded the following results: (a) Thirty-one participants (56%) were classified correctly as lapsers or abstainers by both the telic–paratelic pair and the interaction of the mastery–sympathy pair and version of the autic state; (b) 9 additional participants (16%) were classified correctly by the telic–paratelic pair only; (c) 8 additional participants (14%) were classified correctly only by the interaction of the mastery–sympathy pair with autocentric–intra-autic states; and (d) 8 participants (14%) were incorrectly classified by both the telic–paratelic variable and the interaction. Therefore, 48 participants (86%) were correctly classified as lapsers or abstainers by using the parameters suggested by the logit modeling procedures.

DISCUSSING THE MEANING BEHIND THE RESULTS

The results of this study have important implications for both reversal theory and smoking cessation. The finding that the metamotivational pairs were largely unrelated to each other reflects Apter's contention (e.g., Apter, 1989) that each

Table 2   Frequencies of Participants in Intra-Autic Mastery
and Sympathy States and Autocentric Mastery and Sympathy
States by Lapse Versus Abstain

Smoking outcome	Intra-autic sympathy	Autocentric sympathy	Intra-autic mastery	Autocentric mastery
Lapse	8[a]	3	5	6[a]
Abstain	3	3	25[a]	3

[a]Correct predictions: 39 of 56 (70%).

of the pairs provides a unique contribution to explaining phenomenological experience. Reversal theory constructs represent the richness of the phenomenological field, but they also give a structure to phenomenology. In the case of relapse crises, this structure gives clues to whether an unhealthy addictive behavior will be engaged in. Individuals who are in playful states are more likely to smoke. In addition, people who are oriented to caring for or consoling themselves are likely to succumb to the urge. Also, individuals concerned with mastering others are also likely to lapse. Individuals concerned with mastering others may feel that they need a cigarette to succeed in doing so, whereas individuals concerned with mastering themselves (intra-autic mastery) are more likely to resist smoking. Individuals who are oriented toward mastering or controlling themselves are more likely to resist the urge.

It is worth noting that none of the participants in this data set was coded as alloic. This does not indicate that the alloic state is unnecessary in explaining human behavior. People experiencing relapse crises may be naturally self-centered rather than other-centered at the time of the crisis. In previous work, participants occasionally told the present authors that they smoked in a situation in order to show empathy or camaraderie with another smoker. No such instances appeared in this data set. However, it is possible that the alloic state may be a factor in some lapses.

This study is one of the few that has used all of the reversal theory states in combination to predict a specific outcome. Overall, the model correctly classified 86% of the participants. This percentage compares favorably with the models that contained cigarette availability along with specific pairs of metamotivational states. This illustrates that psychological factors are as important as the presence of the addictive substance in stimulating smoking during a quit attempt. In particular, certain types of metamotivational states are associated with lapsing, and others are associated with resisting the urge to smoke. These findings do not imply that participants should try to prevent themselves from entering certain states. Apter (1989) has claimed that it is normal to experience all the states. Mental health demands it. However, within any particular state there are certain vulnerabilities and certain strengths that need to be recognized and used.

CONCLUSION

Reversal theory suggests that resisting the urge to smoke demands different strategies in different states. For instance, individuals who have urges when they are in the paratelic state are particularly vulnerable to lapsing. Most of the coping strategies used to resist the urge to smoke have a telic orientation. These include thinking about the long-term consequences of smoking and doing relaxation exercises. In the paratelic state, however, the individual is focused on the present moment, not the future, and is looking for arousal, not relaxation. To resist the urge to smoke in the paratelic state, coping strategies that are different from those usually recommended must be used. Cognitive strategies that focus on the immediate aversive effects of smoking and behavioral strategies to increase arousal are examples of coping efforts that are consistent with the preferences of the paratelic state. This study also showed that participants in the intraautic sympathy state are likely to lapse. This state is characterized by feeling deprived and unnurtured. Exhortations to oneself to be strong and to use willpower are entirely inconsistent with what one feels in the intra-autic sympathy state. Focusing on smoking as a method of self-abuse, not self-care, while engaging in other means of self-nurturance are methods that are more consistent with the preferences of the intra-autic sympathy state. This analysis indicates that reversal theory not only has explanatory power with respect to addictive behaviors but also provides solid theoretical underpinnings for improved interventions and better health outcomes.

REFERENCES

Apter, M. J. (1989). *Reversal theory: Motivation, emotion, and personality.* London: Routlege.
Baer, J. S., Lichtenstein, E., Ransom, C. C., & Kamarck, T. (1989). Prediction of smoking relapse: Analysis of temptations and transgressions after initial cessation. *Journal of Consulting and Clinical Psychology, 57,* 623–627.
Bliss, R. E., Garvey, A. J., Heinold, J. W., & Hitchcock, J. L. (1989). The influence of situation and coping on relapse crisis outcomes after smoking cessation. *Journal of Consulting and Clinical Psychology, 57,* 443–449.
Brandon, T. H., Tiffany, S. T., & Baker, T. B. (1986). The process of smoking relapse. In F. M. Tims & C. G. Leukefeld (Eds.), *Relapse and recovery in drug abuse* (Monograph 72, pp. 104–117). Rockville, MD: National Institute on Drug Abuse.
Cohen, J. (1960). A coefficient of agreement for nominal scales. *Educational and Psychological Measurement, 20,* 37–46.
Cook, M. R., Gerkovich, M. M., O'Connell, K., & Potocky, M. (1995). Reversal theory constructs and cigarette availability predict lapse early in smoking cessation. *Research in Nursing & Health, 18,* 217–224.
O'Connell, K. A., Cook, M. R., Gerkovich, M. M., Potocky, M., & Swan, G. E. (1990). Reversal theory and smoking: A state-based approach to ex-smokers' highly tempting situations. *Journal of Consulting and Clinical Psychology, 58,* 489–494.
O'Connell, K., Gerkovich, M. M., & Cook, M. R. (1995). Reversal theory's mastery and sympathy states in smoking cessation. *Image: Journal of Nursing Scholarship, 27,* 311–316.
O'Connell, K. A., & Martin, E. J. (1987). Highly tempting situations associated with abstinence, temporary lapse, and relapse among participants in smoking cessation programs. *Journal of Consulting and Clinical Psychology, 55,* 367–371.
O'Connell, K. A., Potocky, M., Cook, M. R., & Gerkovich, M. M. (1991). *Metamotivational State Interview and Coding Schedule instruction manual.* Kansas City, MO: Midwest Research Institute.
Potocky, M., Gerkovich, M. M., O'Connell, K. A., & Cook, M. R. (1991). State-outcome consistency in smoking relapse crises: A reversal theory approach. *Journal of Consulting and Clinical Psychology, 59,* 351–353.
Shiffman, S. (1986). A cluster-analytic classification of smoking relapse episodes. *Addictive Behaviors, 11,* 295–307.
Shiffman, S. (1993). Smoking cessation treatment: Any progress? *Journal of Consulting and Clinical Psychology, 61,* 718–722.

9

Differential EEG Effects of Smoking in the Telic and Paratelic States

Mary R. Cook, Mary M. Gerkovich, and Kathleen A. O'Connell

Fifty smokers were divided into telic, paratelic, and intermediate dominance groups. Three measures of central nervous system (CNS) activity were each obtained while participants were deprived of smoking, "sham" smoked an unlit cigarette, and smoked. Data were analyzed in terms of both dominance and the state (telic or paratelic) the participant was experiencing at the time of smoking. All three measures yielded significant results relevant to reversal theory concepts. If replicated and extended, these findings should clarify the CNS mechanisms that underlie dominance and state and the way in which gender-specific brain organization relates to reversal theory concepts.

Previous work from the authors' laboratory has confirmed the hypothesis that reversal theory constructs are relevant to smoking and smoking cessation (e.g., Cook, Gerkovich, Hoffman, et al., 1995; Cook, Gerkovich, O'Connell, & Potocky, 1995; O'Connell, Gerkovich, & Cook, 1995; Potocky, Gerkovich, O'Connell, & Cook, 1991; see also Chapter 8 by O'Connell, Gerkovich, and Cook). Arousal and its associated hedonic tone are key concepts in reversal theory and in many models of smoking and smoking cessation. There is extensive evidence that smoking increases CNS arousal (see Gilbert, 1995, for review) and that under certain circumstances smoking can also have arousal-decreasing proper-

The work reported here was supported by Grant NR01675 from the National Institute of Nursing Research, Mary R. Cook, Principal Investigator. The authors wish to thank Steven J. Hoffman, F. Joseph McClernon, and Harvey D. Cohen for their important contributions to the research.

ties (e.g., Cinciripini, 1986; Gilbert, Robinson, Chamberlin, & Spielberger, 1989; Golding & Mangan, 1982). The aim of the work summarized here was to further understand the effects of smoking on measures of CNS arousal and activation from a reversal theory perspective. Because the telic and paratelic modes are defined in terms of arousal and its associated phenomenological experience, the focus was on the telic–paratelic pair, and particularly on the arousal-seeking and arousal-avoidance component of the pair. The overall hypothesis was that, in the telic state, people will smoke in such a way as to decrease arousal, whereas in the paratelic state, people will smoke in such a way as to increase arousal.

Although this hypothesis seems simple and straightforward, it must be pointed out that arousal is not a unitary concept. Pribram and McGuinness (1975) postulated three major arousal regulatory systems: an arousal system that produces a phasic response to perceptual input, an activation system that maintains readiness for action, and an effort system that coordinates the other two. Tucker and Williamson (1984) concluded that the arousal system is adrenergic, with maximal distribution in the right parietal area, and that the activation system is dopaminergic, with maximal distribution in the left frontal area of the brain. Svebak (e.g., Svebak, 1984, 1985) related this model to reversal theory and reported data indicating that the paratelic state is dominated by the arousal system and the telic state is dominated by the activation system.

If the model proposed by Pribram and McGuinness (1975) is correct, and if the activation and arousal systems do in fact underlie the telic and paratelic states, respectively, the following phenomena should be observed.

1   Spectral analysis of the electroencephalogram (EEG; discrete Fourier Transform, or DFT) reflects rapid changes in arousal. The lowest frequency component (Δ, 1–3.75 Hz) is observed during sleep; theta frequencies (4–7.75 Hz) occur during drowsiness and reverie; alert wakefulness is associated with the alpha rhythm (8–12 Hz); and high arousal is reflected in Beta 1 waves (12.25–22 Hz) and Beta 2 waves (22.25–30 Hz). All of these components appear in the waking EEG, and arousal levels are estimated by the relative amplitude or power of each component. It was reasoned that the paratelic state and paratelic dominance would be best reflected by the DFT because it reflects phasic changes in the arousal system.

2   The contingent negative variation (CNV) reflects both orienting (early component) and preparation for action (late component). It is a negative shift in brain potential that occurs between the warning and imperative signals in a fixed-period reaction time task. Because it reflects preparation for goal-directed action, the CNV should best reflect the telic member of the pair.

3   Presentation of a stimulus causes a complex brain response that, when averaged over several stimuli, reflects both sensory processing and information processing (event-related potential, or ERP). The early components reflect sensory processing (a negative shift approximately 100 ms after the stimulus, N100)

and stimulus evaluation (a positive shift approximately 200 ms after the stimulus, P200). Both amplitude and latency measures are used to evaluate the ERP. The early components should be more sensitive to dominance than to state, as the sensory processes are relatively unaffected by cognitive events. In the work reported here, ERP data were obtained during the CNV task.

4 Smoking in the two states should have differential effects on all three of these measures (DFT, CNV, ERP). Smoking in the telic state should result in decreased CNS arousal, and smoking in the paratelic state should result in increased CNS arousal.

5 The relationship between state and dominance has received little empirical attention in reversal theory research (see Chapter 7 by Spicer and Lyons). If state is a more powerful predictor of the effects of smoking than is dominance, it would imply that the underlying mechanism is capable of brief, phasic response; if dominance is the better predictor, it would indicate that hard-wired neural systems form the underlying mechanisms. Both dominance and state analyses were therefore used to test the hypotheses. Although the hypotheses are concerned with the effects of smoking, the results help clarify the biological basis of the telic–paratelic pair.

STUDY METHOD

Participants

Volunteers from the community who had smoked at least a pack a day for the past 2 years were recruited for the study. All were right-handed, as confirmed by the Edinburgh Handedness Inventory (Oldfield, 1971), and in good health. In a screening session, volunteers completed the Paratelic Dominance Scale (PDS; Cook & Gerkovich, 1993) and several personality–trait measures. Those volunteers with PDS scores of 15 to 30 were considered to be paratelic-dominant, those with a score between 0 and 6 were considered to be telic-dominant, and those with a score of 7–14 were considered to be intermediate (i.e., displaying neither telic nor paratelic dominance). From the pool of volunteers, participants were selected so as to form equal numbers of men and women in each of the three dominance groups. The final sample consisted of 50 volunteers (25 men, 25 women) aged 18–52 years ($M = 32$) with a representative proportion of minority volunteers (26%). Participants smoked an average of 26 cigarettes per day and had done so for an average of 14.6 years.

Physiological Recording

The EEG was recorded from Ag–AgCl electrodes at the left frontal (F3), right frontal (F4), central (Cz), left parietal (P3), and right parietal (P4) sites on the scalp (International 10-20 placement system), using commercially prepared electrode gel. Linked mastoids served as reference electrodes, and a ground electrode was placed at middle forehead. The electrooculogram (EOG) was recorded from sites above and at the outer canthus of the left eye to delete eye movement artifact.

Procedures

Each participant participated in one training session and one test session. In the training session, participants were made familiar with all of the tasks and procedures to be used, practiced completing subjective rating scales, and practiced sham smoking. In the test session, carbon monoxide was measured to confirm that the participant had complied with instructions to refrain from smoking for 4 hr, and sensors were attached. Participants then completed a battery of tasks that included a resting, eyes-closed condition for spectral analysis of the EEG (see Cook et al., 1995b, for further details), the go and no-go CNV during which both CNV and ERP data were obtained, and a continuous motor performance task. Each task was performed under three conditions: deprived, after sham smoking own cigarette, and after smoking own cigarette. The Somatic State Questionnaire (Cook, Gerkovich, Potocky, & O'Connell, 1993) was administered before and after each task under each condition, and the arousal-seeking subscale was used to determine state. Although smoking conditions were always presented in the same order, the order of tasks was counterbalanced.

Participants sat in an adjustable office-type chair in a sound-attenuated electrically shielded room. They wore headphones and held a small box with a microswitch for responding to the *go* CNV trials. Tones for the warning (S1) and imperative (S2) stimuli were presented to both ears over the headphones. The warning stimulus, S1, could be a low-pitch tone (400 Hz) or a high-pitch tone (1200 Hz); S2 was the simultaneous generation of both frequencies. All tones were of 50 ms duration with 10 ms rise–fall time. A 100-ms burst of white noise was delivered by the same apparatus to signal an incorrect response. The EOG was monitored during trial collections (250 ms before S1 until S2), and trials were immediately rejected if a 100-μv EOG level was detected. Trials with incorrect responses were also immediately rejected.

Analyses

Spectral, CNV, and ERP data were analyzed by means of analysis of variance for mixed designs (BMDP Statistical Software, Program 4V) with smoking condition (deprived, sham, or smoke), site (Cz, F3, F4, P3, P4), and variables specific to each measure serving as within-subject variables. All reported p values involving repeated measures were corrected (Huynh-Feldt ε) for inflated degrees of freedom. For dominance analyses, comparisons were made between telic- and paratelic-dominant participants; state analyses grouped participants by the state they were in at the time and did not take dominance into account. There was no significant relationship between dominance and state.

Spectral Analysis

Dominance

Smoking increased alpha frequency, an effect that has been reported by many investigators. No differential effects of smoking were found for alpha power or for theta power. However, telic-dominant participants showed decreased Beta 2 power after smoking, whereas paratelic-dominant participants showed increased Beta 2 power; the results were the same for all sites ($p < .05$). Similar but weaker results were found for Beta 1 power. The dominance results support the hypothesis that telic-dominant people will smoke in such a way as to decrease arousal and paratelic-dominant people will smoke in such a way as to increase arousal.

State

As shown in Figure 1, smoking in the telic state decreased theta power; smoking in the paratelic state did not alter it ($p = .02$). Telic participants showed no change in either alpha or beta power, indicating that the decrease in theta power was associated with a shift of power into the lower frequency delta component

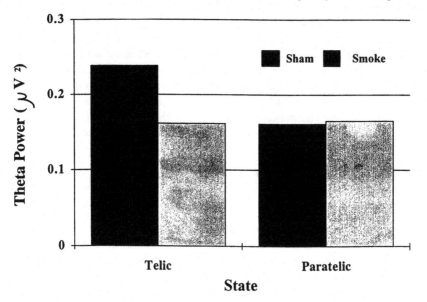

Figure 1 Smoking decreases theta power in participants in the telic state but does not alter it in participants in the paratelic state. Because no increases in alpha power were observed, the results are interpreted as supporting the hypothesis that participants in the telic state will smoke in such a way as to decrease CNS arousal.

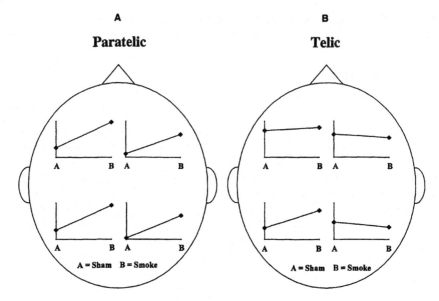

Figure 2 Smoking increases Beta 2 power in participants in the paratelic state but has little effect on Beta 2 power in telic participants.

(i.e., decreased arousal). In contrast, as shown in Figure 2, smoking in the paratelic state significantly increased Beta 2 power at all sites, whereas smoking in the telic state had little or no effect ($p = .03$). The results indicate that, as expected, smoking in the telic state decreases measures of CNS arousal (shift to lower frequencies), whereas smoking in the paratelic state increases CNS arousal (shift to higher frequencies). Spectral analysis had been expected to be more sensitive to paratelic dominance and state than to telic dominance and state. The results were more complex and indicate that changes in theta power better reflect telic processes and changes in beta power better reflect paratelic processes.

CONTINGENT NEGATIVE VARIATION

Dominance

As expected, the go CNV was larger than the no-go CNV (e.g., at Cz, $p < .001$). The shape of the overall CNV differed for telic- and paratelic-dominant participants. The CNV was larger for telic than for paratelic participants during the early, orienting part of the interstimulus interval; the CNV amplitude at the end of the interval, which reflects action readiness, was larger for paratelic than for telic participants. The effect was significant at Cz ($p = .05$) and P3 ($p = .03$); a trend was observed at P4 ($p = .09$). Figure 3 shows the data from CZ. The results are consistent with reversal theory constructs; telic-dominant people tend

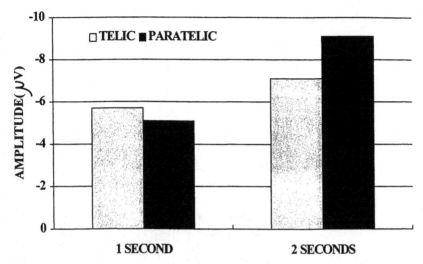

Figure 3 The pattern of the contingent negative variation is different for telic- and paratelic-dominant participants. Telic-dominant participants show larger response 1 s after the warning stimulus, and paratelic-dominant participants show a larger response just before the imperative stimulus.

to prepare for action soon after being warned that action will be required; paratelic-dominant people tend to prepare just before the imperative stimulus.

Consistent with the general literature on smoking and the CNV, smoking increased CNV amplitude at parietal and vertex sites, but did not significantly affect the CNV at frontal sites. Differential effects of smoking on telic- and paratelic-dominant participants were found as a function of gender for the no-go CNV, but not for the go CNV. This complicated interaction indicates that an imperative need to perform quickly and accurately dissipates dominance differences in the effects of smoking. Significant Dominance Group × Gender × Smoking Condition interactions were found at Cz ($p = .02$) and at P3 ($p = .03$); a trend was found at P4 ($p = .06$). The results are summarized in Figure 4. Figure 4A shows the data for men; Figure 4B shows the data for women. The units shown are the absolute difference in CNV amplitude between the sham-smoking period and the smoking period. It appears that the primary source of this interaction is the differences between men and women in the differential effects of smoking on telic- and paratelic-dominant people. For men, the differential smoking effects were as hypothesized: Smoking increased the early, orienting component of no-go CNV at all sites for telic-dominant men and had little effect on the later, action readiness component of the no-go CNV; for paratelic-dominant men, however, smoking had a larger effect on the late action-readiness component of the no-go CNV than on the early orienting component. Smoking had differential effects for telic- and paratelic-dominant women; these smoking-induced changes, however, were different from those observed in men and were very unexpected. Smoking decreased both the early and late components of the CNV in telic-

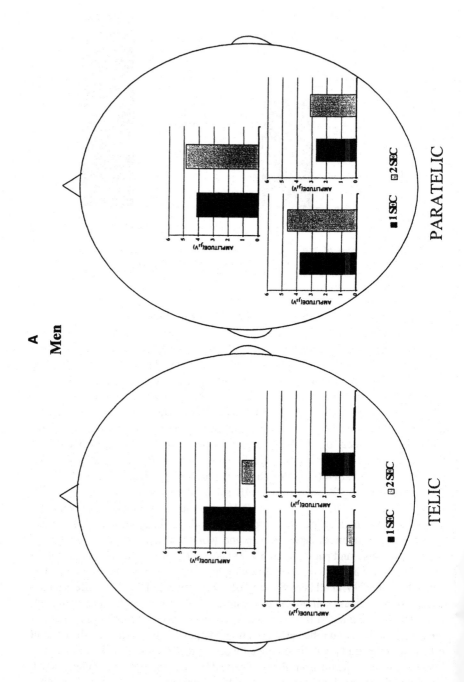

A
Men

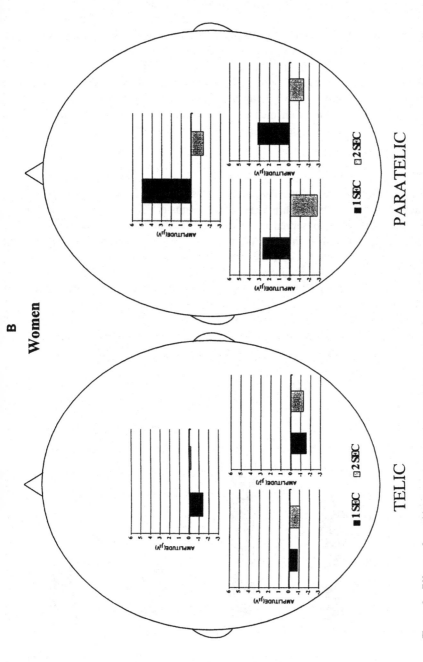

Figure 4 Effects of smoking on no-go contingent negative variation amplitude for men (A) and women (B). The units shown are the differences between sham and smoking conditions. Data are shown for central, left parietal, and right parietal sites.

111

dominant women; this result is counter to the general findings in the literature that smoking increases CNV amplitude. The smoking-induced changes for paratelic-dominant women, however, were different from those seen in both paratelic-dominant men and telic-dominant women. Consistent with findings reported in the literature, smoking increased the early component of the CNV for paratelic-dominant women. Smoking, however, decreased the later, action-readiness component of the CNV in paratelic-dominant women. The smoking-induced changes in women did not support the hypothesis. These results do, however, point to the importance of including both men and women in studies of the physiological implications of telic and paratelic dominance.

State

The CNV pattern for go and no-go tasks was different for participants in the paratelic and telic states. Figure 5 shows the results at F3 ($p = .029$); a trend for the same pattern was observed at F4 ($p = .054$). Participants in the telic state had larger go CNV than those in the paratelic state during both the early and late components of the CNV. This pattern was also found for the early component of the no-go CNV. In contrast, participants in the paratelic state had larger late component no-go CNV than participants in the telic state. Although the overall shape of the CNV was different in the telic and paratelic states, smoking did not differentially alter the CNV as a function of state.

Overall, the CNV results showed that smoking differentially altered the CNV in the dominance analysis, but not in the state analysis. In the dominance

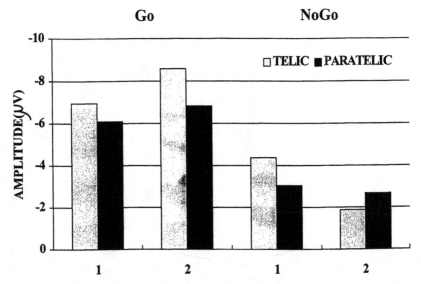

Figure 5   Differences in the shape of the go and no-go contingent negative variation as a function of whether the participants were in the telic or paratelic state.

analysis, telic participants showed an advantage (larger CNV amplitude) over the paratelic participants in the early, orienting component of the CNV; the paratelic participants, however, had increased amplitude during the late, action-readiness component of the CNV. This same pattern was seen with the no-go stimuli in the state analysis; telic participants had larger early CNV amplitude compared with paratelic participants, whereas paratelic participants had larger late CNV amplitude. For the go stimuli, telic participants showed larger amplitude than paratelic participants during both the early and late components of the CNV. In addition, pervasive interactions with gender were found for dominance groups, but not when participants were divided by state. Further research using alternative CNV techniques is needed to clarify the extent to which CNV is a good outcome measure for reversal theory research.

EVENT-RELATED POTENTIAL

Dominance

It was expected that smoking-induced changes in the early components of ERP would be more sensitive to dominance than to state differences. The N100 amplitude, which reflects sensory processing, was increased by smoking at all sites for paratelic-dominant participants; telic-dominant participants showed little change in N100 amplitude as a function of smoking (Cz, $p = .012$; F3, $p = .03$; F4, $p = .017$; P3, $p = .011$; P4, $p = .026$). In contrast, the amplitude of the P200 component, which reflects stimulus evaluation, was significantly decreased by smoking for paratelic-dominant participants, but not for telic-dominant participants at Cz ($p = .022$) and P3 ($p = .022$). The results are summarized in Figure 6. Although some trends related to dominance group were found for N100 and P200 latency, none reached statistical significance. The results indicate that ERP data from paratelic-dominant participants, but not from telic-dominant participants, reflected the expected smoking-induced changes in both the N100 and P200 amplitude measures.

State

When ERP data were analyzed on the basis of state groupings, smoking increased both N100 and P200 amplitude at all sites. Differential effects by state were found for N100 amplitude; participants in the paratelic state had greater N100 amplitude than telic participants at Cz ($p = .046$), F3 ($p = .014$), F4 ($p = .031$), and P3 ($p = .088$). There were no differential effects of smoking on ERP amplitude due to state; N100 was greater for paratelic participants both before and after smoking. The N100 and P200 latencies differed by state and gender, unlike the dominance analysis, which found no differences due to dominance. Telic men had faster N100 than telic women, and paratelic women had faster N100 than paratelic men. This was observed at all sites (Cz, $p = .001$; F3, $p = $

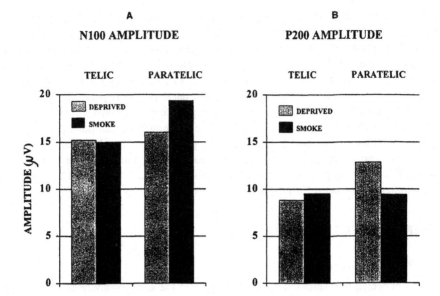

Figure 6 Changes in N100 and P200 event-related potential amplitude for telic- and paratelic-dominant participants. N100 = negative shift approximately 100 ms after the stimulus; P200 = positive shift approximately 200 ms after the stimulus.

.003; F4, $p = .002$; P3, $p = .002$; P4, $p = .006$). The P200 latency differences for men and women in the telic and paratelic states were also found, but were not as symmetrical as the N100 results. Like the N100 results, paratelic women had faster P200 than paratelic men; there were, however, no gender differences for telic participants (F3, $p = .01$; F4, $p = .034$; P3, $p = .019$; P4, $p = .051$). Differential effects of smoking as a function of state were not observed for either N100 or P200 latency.

CONCLUSION

Three different measures of CNS arousal were taken while smokers were deprived of smoking, sham-smoked an unlit cigarette, and smoked a cigarette of their usual brand. Participants were divided into groups in two ways: by scores on the PDS and by the state they were in at the time as determined by the Arousal-Seeking subscale of the Somatic State Questionnaire. The overall hypothesis was that telic smoking results in decreased CNS arousal and paratelic smoking results in increased CNS arousal.

The hypothesis that telic people would smoke in such a way as to decrease arousal and paratelic people would smoke in such a way as to increase arousal was clearly supported for both state and dominance when spectral analysis of the EEG was used as the measure of CNS activity. Theta power best reflected the effects of telic smoking, and Beta 2 power best reflected the effects of paratelic smoking. The spectral data were expected to be most sensitive to paratelic state and dominance because of the phasic nature of the DFT, but instead it was found that changes in the EEG occurred in different frequency components for telic and paratelic smoking.

Smoking differentially altered both CNV and ERP data when participants were divided by dominance groups, but not when they were divided by the state they were experiencing at the time. Furthermore, the CNV of men and women after smoking was quite different for telic- and paratelic-dominant participants, indicating that the brain mechanisms underlying dominance might be different in men and women.

The CNV differentiated between telic and paratelic groups. Telic-dominant participants and those in the telic state showed negative brain potential shifts earlier than paratelic-dominant participants or those in the paratelic state. This finding is consistent with reversal theory descriptions of the telic–paratelic pair. The hypothesis that the CNV would be more sensitive to the telic state than the paratelic state was not supported.

ERP amplitude, as expected, reflected dominance better than state. No significant effects of smoking were found when participants were divided into groups on the basis of the state they were in when they smoked. The state data did, however, yield some intriguing and unexpected results. Amplitude of the N100 component of the ERP was larger for paratelic- than telic-dominant participants both before and after smoking. Latency of N100 and P200 interacted with both gender and state, indicating that CNS mechanisms underlying state may be different in men and women.

This is, to the authors' knowledge, the first psychophysiological study of smoking that used reversal theory concepts. It is important that the results be replicated and extended and that the concept of tension-stress be incorporated into further research of this type. It is also important to further consider the implications for reversal theory research of the many differences found between men and women and to determine whether these differences would be obtained for a sample of nonsmokers. Psychophysiological studies of reversal theory have previously been shown by Svebak and his colleagues to be important to a better understanding of the mechanisms that underlie dominance and state in the telic–paratelic pair (e.g., see review by Apter & Svebak, 1992). Reversal theory has also been shown to be very relevant to smoking and smoking cessation. It is therefore important to continue research that combines these two approaches.

REFERENCES

Apter, M. J., & Sveback, S. (1992). Reversal theory as a biological approach to individual differences. In A. Gale & M. W. Eysenck (Eds.), *Handbook of individual differences: Biological perspectives* (pp. 323–353). New York: Wiley.

Cinciripini, P. M. (1986). The effects of smoking and electrocortical arousal in coronary prone (Type A) and non-coronary prone (Type B) subjects. *Psychopharmacology, 90*, 522–527.

Cook, M. R., & Gerkovich, M. M. (1993). The development of a paratelic dominance scale. In J. H. Kerr, S. Murgatroyd, & M. J. Apter (Eds.), *Advances in reversal theory* (pp. 177–188). Amsterdam: Swets & Zeitlinger.

Cook, M. R., Gerkovich, M. M., Hoffman, S. J., McClernon, F. J., Cohen, H. D., Oakleaf, K. L., & O'Connell, K. A. (1995). Smoking and EEG power spectra: Effects of differences in arousal seeking. *International Journal of Psychophysiology, 19,* 247–256.

Cook, M. R., Gerkovich, M. M., O'Connell, K. A., & Potocky, M. (1995). Reversal theory constructs and cigarette availability predict lapse in early smoking cessation. *Research in Nursing and Health, 18,* 217–224.

Cook, M. R., Gerkovich, M. M., Potocky, M., & O'Connell, K. A. (1993). Instruments for the assessment of reversal theory states. *Patient Education and Counseling, 22,* 99–106.

Gilbert, D. G. (1995). *Smoking: Individual differences, psychopathology, and emotion.* Washington, DC: Taylor & Francis.

Gilbert, D. G., Robinson, J. H., Chamberlin, C. L., & Spielberger, C. D. (1989). Effects of smoking/nicotine on lateralization of EEG while viewing a stressful move. *Psychophysiology, 26,* 311–320.

Golding, J., & Mangan, G. L. (1982). Arousing and de-arousing effects of cigarette smoking under conditions of stress and mild sensory deprivation. *Psychophysiology, 19,* 449–456.

O'Connell, K. A., Cook, M. R., Gerkovich, M. M., Potocky, M., & Swan, G. E. (1990). Reversal theory and smoking: A state-based approach to ex-smokers' highly tempting situations. *Journal of Consulting and Clinical Psychology, 58,* 489–494.

O'Connell, K. A., Gerkovich, M. M., & Cook, M. R. (1995). Reversal theory's mastery and sympathy states in smoking cessation. *Image: Journal of Nursing Scholarship, 27,* 311–316.

Oldfield, R. C. (1971). The assessment and analysis of handedness: The Edinburgh Inventory. *Neuropsychologia, 9,* 97–113.

Pribram, K., & McGuinness, D. (1975). Arousal, activation and effort in the control of attention. *Psychological Review, 82,* 116–149

Potocky, M., Gerkovich, M. M., O'Connell, K. A., & Cook, M. R. (1991). State-outcome consistency in smoking relapse crises: A reversal theory approach. *Journal of Consulting and Clinical Psychology, 59,* 351–353.

Svebak, S. (1984). Active and passive forearm flexor tension patterns in the continuous perceptual-motor task paradigm: The significance of motivation. *International Journal of Psychophysiology, 2,* 167–176.

Svebak, S. (1985). Serious-mindedness and the effect of self-induced respiratory changes upon parietal EEG. *Biofeedback and Self-Regulation, 10,* 49–62.

Tucker, D. M., & Williamson, P. A. (1984). Asymmetric neural control systems in human self-regulations. *Psychological Review, 91,* 185–215.

IV

RISK-TAKING BEHAVIOR

10

Gratuitous Risk:
A Study of Parachuting

Michael J. Apter and Robert Batler

Reversal theory suggests that many kinds of potentially self-damaging behavior (so-called "paradoxical behavior") can be understood as involving deliberate exposure to risk, with the aim of achieving excitement. The theory posits that the typical way in which this occurs is that the danger increases arousal levels in the telic state, producing anxiety, and then mastery of the danger triggers a reversal to the paratelic state in which the high arousal is enjoyed instead as excitement. In the present study, a particular form of gratuitous risk—that of sport parachuting— was studied by means of questionnaire. The responses showed that, consistent with the reversal theory prediction, anxiety was most prevalent just before the perceived moment of maximum danger and excitement was most prevalent just after this moment. Respondents also indicated that excitement-seeking was the main reason for their practice of the sport, although satisfactions relating to all the metamotivational states were cited in different combinations by different respondents.

THE PURSUIT OF EXCITEMENT

One of the strengths of reversal theory is that it provides explanations for what might be termed "paradoxical behavior" (Apter, 1982). This is defined as behavior that is voluntarily undertaken and yet that appears to militate against

Our sincere thanks are due to the administration of Parachute Associates of Indiana and Hinckley Parachute Center, Inc., of Illinois, both for their permission to allow us to administer these questionnaires to their members and for their help in implementing this process. We are also grateful to the respondents in both clubs for their freely given time. In addition, we wish to acknowledge the invaluable help of Mr. Young Kim at the University of Chicago, who collected data as part of the pilot study of the questionnaire used here. We should also like to record our condolences to the family and friends of Mr. Ron Harris, one of our participants, who was killed in an airplane crash shortly after our study was completed.

119

the health, well-being, and even survival of the individual concerned, exposing him or her to gratuitous risk (see Chapter 2). It may take many forms (Kerr & Apter, 1991; Kerr, Frank-Ragan, & Brown, 1993). For example, why do people damage their health by smoking? Why do people persist in risky sexual behavior in the age of AIDS? Why do people often drive faster than they need to?

The particular kind of paradoxical behavior that is the subject of this chapter is that of dangerous sport. This involves deliberately confronting oneself with physical danger and is exemplified by such activities as mountaineering, extreme skiing, white-water rafting, hang-gliding, bungee-jumping, pot-holing, and deep-sea diving. Dangerous sport may also be said to relate to such psychologically similar, if less institutionalized, risky street sports as elevator and underground train surfing and soccer hooliganism (Kerr, 1994), as well as an ever-shifting range of teenage fads and cults. Clearly, all these kinds of risky activity are likely to be performed by people who are more sensation-seeking than others (Zuckerman, 1979), and, consistent with this, there is evidence from work using the Telic Dominance Scale that they are also more paratelic-dominant (Chirivella & Martinez, 1994; Kerr, 1991; Kerr & Svebak, 1989). The focus of this chapter, however, is not enduring personality characteristics, but the actor-in-the-situation, over the relatively short period of time involved in the risk-taking activity itself.

Such gratuitously risky activities have been analyzed at length from the reversal theory perspective in a book titled *The Dangerous Edge*, which also includes explorations of a variety of other excitement-seeking behaviors that are not in themselves risky, such as watching horror movies (Apter, 1992). One of the basic ideas of this book is that by confronting oneself with genuinely dangerous situations, the individual manages to create a high level of arousal in himself or herself. This arousal is likely, initially, to be experienced in the telic state as anxiety. But then at some point the danger is overcome (re-establishing what can be termed a *protective frame* in the individual's experience), and the paratelic state returns, converting the anxiety to excitement. For the activity as a whole to be worthwhile, the excitement gained in this way must be enjoyed for a longer period than the anxiety, so that, taken overall, the pleasure outweighs the displeasure.

It may be helpful to think of this sequence in terms of Figure 1A in Chapter 1. Here one can visualize the individual's arousal increasing down the telic curve and becoming increasingly unpleasant (anxiety), and then, when reversal occurs, jumping up to the point vertically above on the paratelic curve so that the high arousal is now experienced as pleasant (excitement). It can be seen that the greater the anxiety before the reversal, the greater the excitement that immediately follows it. High anxiety, in this manner, can give rise to such emotions as euphoria and even ecstasy. This explanatory account is consistent with Zillmann's (1984) demonstration of *excitation-transfer* from one emotion to another, but adds to it the emotional structure of the telic and paratelic states and the notion of reversal between them.

For the study that is described in this chapter, it was decided to research the experience of dangerous sport by means of a questionnaire. This questionnaire was subjected to a trial run with people engaged in a range of dangerous sports (including river rafting, scuba diving, and cliff scaling) and then rewritten to avoid, as far as possible, ambiguities, redundancies, and other infelicities.

The primary aim of the study was to see if the anxiety-to-excitement phenomenon posited in reversal theory could indeed be discerned in dangerous sports. In other words, do people tend to experience their maximum anxiety in such activities just before moments in which they perceive great danger and experience their maximum excitement immediately following such moments, when the danger has been mastered? Parachuting was chosen as the particular sport for study because of the simplicity of its temporal structure; that is, in the normal way of things, and for any one trial, there is one particular moment where the reversal is most likely to take effect. In other words, there is a clear-cut moment of maximum danger: the moment between jumping out of the aircraft and the opening of the parachute. (So as not to prejudge the issue, however, the respondents in this study were allowed to designate what was for them their own moment of maximum danger and to answer the relevant questions in terms of this precise moment.) It will be realized that parachuting contrasts in terms of this dramatic simplicity with most other dangerous sports, like mountain climbing, where heightened danger may occur at almost any moment over an extended period of time, often unexpectedly. Parachuting has been used before because of its convenience in this respect for the empirical study of emotions that relate to stress. Notable here is the work of Epstein (1967) and Fenz and Epstein (1967), although their research emphasized the emotions of fear and anxiety and the way that these negative emotions are handled.

A second aim of the research was to look at all the different satisfactions that sports parachuting might provide, taking into account the full set of metamotivational modes. In other words, although it was expected that the main satisfaction would be likely to be paratelic excitement, it was also of interest to see what other pleasures might be generated by the activity. As would seem to be the case in many voluntarily chosen activities, it was expected that a number of satisfactions (and therefore metamotivational states) might be involved in different aspects of the activity at the same or at different times.

Questions were also included in the questionnaire to find out more about the respondents and to probe a little further into the way in which they experienced their sport.

RESEARCH METHOD: THE QUESTIONNAIRE

Participants

Participants ($N = 61$) were members of two parachute clubs based in the Chicago area: Parachute Associates of Frankfurt, Indiana ($n = 46$), and Hinckley Parachute Center, Inc., of Hinckley, Illinois ($n = 15$). Their participation was voluntary.

Instrument

The data collection instrument was a questionnaire consisting of the 12 questions listed in the box below:

1 Name of dangerous sport:
2 At what level do you practice this sport?
   Professional
   Advanced amateur
   Inexperienced amateur
   Beginner or one-time participant
3 How long have you been practicing it?
4 Are there dangerous sports that you enjoy other than the one specified above?
5 Are there any dangerous sports that you would never engage in under any circumstances?
6 What would you say is the nature of the pleasure that you derive from this sport? (Check all such pleasures or pleasurable feelings.)
   a Serious achievement
   b Immediate fun
   c Relief afterwards
   d Excitement or thrill
   e Defying convention
   f Being part of a community of group
   g Control and mastery
   h Being a center of concerned attention
   i Helping others master the situation
   j Being concerned for others
   k Other (please describe)
7 If you checked more than one of the pleasures listed, please select the letter corresponding to the greatest pleasure for you (the pleasure that you consider more than any other).
8 In your experience is the danger
   a Something that is enjoyed in itself?
   b Something that is endured to gain pleasure from other aspects of the situation?
   Please check one of the above.
9 In practicing the sport, what do you experience as the most important thing protecting you from danger? (Check one from the list below):
   a Your own skill and knowledge
   b The skill and knowledge of others
   c Protective clothing or equipment
   d God, fate, or luck
   e Other (please specify)

10 In the normal course of the activity (i.e., excluding exceptional or unforeseen circumstances), what does the moment of maximum danger consist of?

11 What is the worst thing that could happen to you if everything went wrong?

12 In the diagram, the moment of maximum danger is represented on a time dimension, with minutes before represented by negative numbers and minutes afterward by positive numbers. On this diagram, please do the following:

    a If you feel fear or anxiety at any time during the whole period indicated, show when it is at its maximum, by means of an X in the appropriate segment, and write an A above it.

    b Do likewise for excitement or thrill, marking it with an E above the X.

    c Finally, if the period of maximum anxiety or excitement falls outside the time period of the diagram, please indicate when such period(s) may occur.

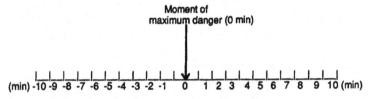

Respondents were also asked to give their name, age, sex, and occupation and to sign a consent form.

Procedure

One hundred copies of this questionnaire were left with Parachute Associates of Frankfurt, Indiana, together with stamped envelopes addressed to the investigators. Forty-six of these questionnaires were voluntarily completed and returned by members of the club. Fifteen other individuals were handed the questionnaire in person at Hinckley Parachutes, Inc., after they had just made a jump, and all of them completed the questionnaire at that time.

CHARACTERISTICS OF THE SAMPLE

Of the sample of 61 individuals, 10 (approximately 16%) were female, and 51 (approximately 84%) were male. The average age was 33.66 years (SD = 9.82 years, range = 18–63). Occupations varied widely and included sales representative, systems analyst, policeman, teacher, electrician, truck driver, and so forth. The average length of time that the participants had been engaged in the sport

(Item 3) was 4.66 years (*SD* = 5.59 years, range = 1 day to 20 years). In terms of level of experience (Item 2), 8 (approximately 13%) described themselves as professional, 12 (approximately 20%) as advanced amateur, 25 (approximately 41%) as experienced amateur, 10 (approximately 16%) as inexperienced amateur, and 6 (approximately 10%) as beginner or one-time participant. The modal response was therefore that of experienced amateur. A majority, 33 (approximately 54%), reported participating in at least one other dangerous sport (Item 4). Two individuals reported as many as six other dangerous sports, but most of these multisport respondents (14, or approximately 23% of the total sample) reported only one other dangerous sport. A majority, 36 (approximately 59%), responded that there were no dangerous sports that they could not conceive of engaging in (Item 5).

REASONS FOR PARTICIPATION

All of the reasons for participating (i.e., pleasures to be derived from the sport as listed in Item 6) were checked by different participants. The most frequently checked, as had been expected, was excitement or thrill (d) with 56 citations. The next most frequent was immediate fun (b) with 51 citations. The order thereafter was serious achievement (a) with 45 citations; control and mastery (g) with 42 citations; being part of a community or group (f), which also had 42 citations; helping others master the situation (i) with 22 citations; defying convention (e) with 19 citations; relief afterward (c) with 15 citations; being concerned for others (j) with 10 citations; and finally being a center of concerned attention (h) with 6 citations. In totaling these responses, it must be remembered that different participants were able to check as many of the reasons given as they wished to. Some participants checked only 1 reason, some checked all 10. The modal number of checks per participant was 4.

Participants were also asked, in Item 7, to nominate the single reason for participating that gave the greatest pleasure. The responses are shown in percentage form in the histogram in Figure 1, in which the reasons are described in terms of the technical language of reversal theory as described in Chapter 1. (The order from top to bottom corresponds to the sequence of responses listed in Item 6 of the questionnaire.) Again, excitement-seeking comes out as easily the most prevalent reason for parachuting, with the mastery motive a distant second.

Because the contribution to the tally per participant is equal across participants in relation to Item 7 (unlike Item 6), it is possible to carry out a chi-square analysis of the distribution. This shows that the null hypothesis must be rejected, $\chi^2(9, N = 61) = 120.21, p < .001$.

Although the excitement-seeking motive proved, not surprisingly, to be the most popular one, all the different basic motives as outlined in reversal theory were nevertheless represented. The data here, as in Chapter 12 of this book, add support to one of the basic tenets of reversal theory, which is that almost any

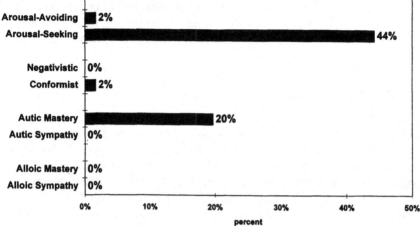

Figure 1 The percentage of participants endorsing, as their primary reason for parachuting, statements representing different basic motives.

activity can be performed to satisfy different motives (in different people or even in the same person at the same or different times).

In responding to Item 6, 15 participants chose to write something in the *other* space. However, there was no compelling evidence for other basic motives that would need to be added to the reversal theory list. Most of the entries were either reformulations of one or another of the motives already posited in the theory (e.g., *adrenaline rush* for *excitement/thrill* and *serenity* for *relief afterwards)* or simply synonyms for pleasure (e.g., *self-satisfaction).* The few exceptions were descriptions of the sensations involved in the activity itself (e.g., sense of flying, experience of free-fall), which could be assimilated to the paratelic desire for intense experiences, and a couple of general statements (*privileged, spiritual experience)* that would need further explication.

PERCEPTION OF THE SITUATION

Not surprisingly, all except 3 participants gave *death* as their response to the question "What is the worst thing that could happen to you if everything went wrong?" (Item 11), the remaining 3 giving permanent injury. (In fact, 6 of the participants giving death as a response also gave injury.) One participant added *death to another,* and 1 participant added getting his family sued for damage caused.

As far as protection from this danger was concerned (the protective frame), 48 respondents (approximately 79% of the sample), checked Item 9a "Your own skill and knowledge." Of the remainder, the majority checked (c), "Protective clothing or equipment."

In response to Item 8, the majority of participants (38, or approximately 63% of the sample) reported that the danger was something to be endured to gain pleasure from other aspects of the situation (Response b) rather than something to be enjoyed in itself (Response a).

ANXIETY-TO-EXCITEMENT REVERSALS

In this part of the analysis, 6 participants had to be excluded because their answer to Item 10, where they were asked to define the moment of maximum danger, was not one that could be meaningfully used in terms of a temporal analysis of subjective feelings before and after that moment. In three cases, the respondents defined the moment of maximum danger in the conditional terms of what would happen if the chute did not open or if they collided with another parachutist, something they had not themselves ever experienced. One participant gave a type of jump, that is, at night. One participant denied that there was any danger at any moment. (In addition, another 5 participants had to be excluded because they did not complete this part of the form.) The following analysis relates to the remaining 50 participants.

The moment judged to be that of maximum danger (Item 10) varied a little from participant to participant, but always fell between the period of leaving the aircraft and the canopy opening. The anxiety and excitement judgments that each participant was asked to make were then made in terms of his or her own personal decision about precisely when this moment of maximum danger occurred.

The histogram shown in Figure 2 indicates for each minute before and after the moment of perceived maximum danger the number of respondents who chose this minute as representing the moment of their maximum anxiety. (Eight participants who denied experiencing any anxiety at any point are not included in the figure.) It will be seen on inspecting this figure that the modal moment for greatest anxiety was that immediately preceding the moment judged to be that of maximum danger, as predicted by reversal theory.

In Figure 3, the histogram is of the same type as that shown in Figure 2, but this time the judgments relate to the moment of maximum excitement rather than to the moment of maximum anxiety. (In this case, 3 participants who indicated that they experienced excitement over the whole period and were unable to choose a point of maximum excitement were excluded from the analysis. A further 3 participants indicated a bracket of time for maximum excitement, and for purposes of analysis they were assigned the point that fell at the center of this range.) It will be seen that the modal moment for maximum excitement was, as predicted, that immediately following the moment of maximum danger. This

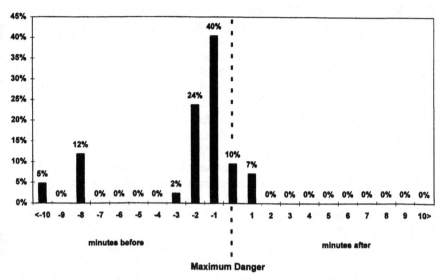

Figure 2 The percentage of participants indicating the moment at which they experienced maximum anxiety, for each minute before or after the moment of perceived maximum danger.

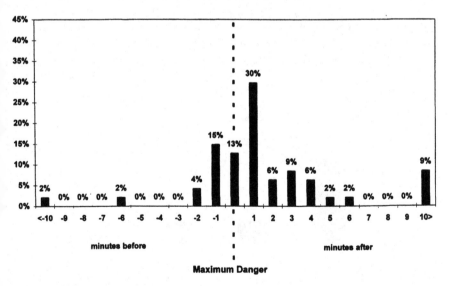

Figure 3 The percentage of participants indicating the moment at which they experienced maximum excitement, for each minute before or after the moment of perceived maximum danger.

way in which anxiety and excitement judgments peak respectively just before and after the maximum danger point is the key finding of this study, demonstrating that for many people one emotion becomes transformed almost instantaneously into the other as the perceived danger itself peaks and disappears.

Because "the moment of maximum danger" is necessarily ambiguous—it is the moment of greatest threat but also the moment at which the threat did not materialize—one might expect some respondents to judge maximum anxiety to occur at this point and some to judge that they experienced maximum excitement at this same point, which is what in fact occurs.

An interesting aspect of these distributions is the way in which, although the modes are so close to each other, the distributions themselves are spread differently over the time range, as can be seen clearly by comparing Figures 2 and 3. A Wilcoxon matched-pairs signed-ranks test showed that participants' time judgments overall were, as would be expected in reversal theory terms, later for maximum excitement judgments than they were for maximum anxiety judgments ($z = 4.9$, $p < .001$, two-tailed).

Another way of looking at all this change-of-emotion data is to ask how many of the participants conformed to the hypothesis that maximum anxiety would occur before, or at, the moment of greatest danger and that maximum excitement would occur at, or following, this moment. This pattern was, in fact, displayed by a majority (30 out of 50) of the participants. To this can be added a further 8 participants who displayed the expected anxiety-to-excitement reversal, although they did not do so around the moment of maximum danger. In another 8 participants, no anxiety was reported, and so the analysis could not be applied to them. (This included the 3 participants who reported being excited during the whole period and were unable to choose a point of maximum excitement.) The only participants whose record showed a pattern directly contrary to the hypothesis were 4 who reported an excitement-to-anxiety reversal. This is all shown in graphical form in Figure 4. On the whole, then, these data sustain the reversal theory account.

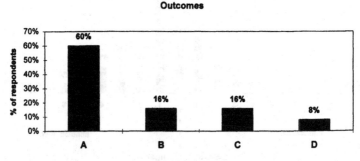

Figure 4 The percentage of participants whose pattern of response corresponded to each of the four possible outcomes listed. A = conforms to hypothesis; B = anxiety–excitement reversal, but not at moment of maximum danger; C = no anxiety reported; D = anxiety–excitement experienced in inverse order.

CONCLUSION

For various reasons that were explored in *The Dangerous Edge* (Apter, 1992), gratuitous risk-seeking would appear to be an inherent part of human nature that, over an evolutionary period, has proved itself to be advantageous to the human species. At the level of the individual, however, especially in modern society, it can lead to a number of health and other kinds of problems that are also discussed in that book. This chapter has been intended as a contribution to an understanding of the basic psychology of this phenomenon of freely chosen risk, through an empirical study of the experience of one representative version of it. One can conclude that the data largely support the reversal theory explanation in terms of anxiety-to-excitement reversals.

REFERENCES

Apter, M. J. (1982). *The experience of motivation: The theory of psychological reversals*. London: Academic Press.

Apter, M. J. (1992). *The dangerous edge: The psychology of excitement*. New York: The Free Press.

Chirivella, E. C., & Martinez, L. M. (1994). The sensation of risk and motivational tendencies in sports: An empirical study. *Personality and Individual Differences, 16,* 777–786.

Epstein, S. (1967). Toward a unified theory of anxiety. In B.A. Maher (Ed.), *Progress in experimental personality research* (Vol. 4, pp. 1–89). New York: Academic Press.

Fenz, W. D., & Epstein, S. (1967). Gradients of physiological arousal, skin conductance, heart rate, and respiration rate as a function of experience. *Psychosomatic Medicine, 29,* 33–51.

Kerr, J. H. (1991). Arousal-seeking in risk sport participants. *Personality and Individual Differences, 12,* 613–616.

Kerr, J. H. (1994). *Understanding soccer hooliganism*. Buckingham, England: Open University Press.

Kerr, J. H., & Apter, M. J. (1991). *Adult play: A reversal theory approach*. Amsterdam: Swets & Zeitlinger.

Kerr, J. H., Frank-Ragan, E., & Brown, R. I. F. (1993). Taking risks with health. *Patient Education and Counselling, 22,* 73–80.

Kerr, J. H., & Svebak, S. (1989). Motivational aspects of preference for, and participation in, "risk" and "safe" sports. *Personality and Individual Differences, 10,* 797–800.

Zillmann, D. (1984). *Connections between sex and aggression*. Hillsdale, NJ: Erlbaum.

Zuckerman, M. (1979). *Sensation seeking: Beyond the optimal level of arousal*. Hillsdale, NJ: Erlbaum.

11

Understanding Sexual Risk-Taking Behavior

Mary M. Gerkovich

Health behavior research continues to focus on why people behave in ways that put their health and lives at risk. An example of this paradox is sexual risk-taking behavior, which puts individuals at risk of HIV infection and the development of AIDS. Much of the research has focused on understanding and changing risk behavior among homosexual men. Research has begun to focus on sexual risk behavior among heterosexual people, as they are the population with the fastest increase in rate of new HIV infection. Traditional models of health behavior have been applied to sexual risk-taking behavior among heterosexual people with only modest success. What is needed is a model that takes into account concepts of reversal theory in order to understand the paradoxes inherent in continued risk behavior by people who are knowledgeable about the risks of HIV infection. A model is proposed that identifies the reversal theory construct of paratelic dominance as an influence on the extent to which people perceive risk in their relationships and have feelings of personal vulnerability, as well as influencing other situational, cognitive, and emotional mediators of condom use. Preliminary support of some of the hypothesized relations is presented.

Most of the health concerns that are the target of current research are the result of actions that run counter to people's own best interests. Sexual risk-taking behavior is an example of this type of paradox: People continue to put their health and lives at risk by not following simple precautionary measures such as using condoms. Much research has documented this health risk, and theories of health behavior have been tested with mixed results. This chapter briefly reviews the literature on sexual risk-taking behavior, reviews the reversal theory concepts that are relevant to sexual risk-taking behavior, and proposes a model that incorporates reversal theory concepts in an attempt to explain why heterosexual people choose to use or not use condoms.

REPORTED RESEARCH EFFORTS

Much research has been carried out on sexual risk-taking behavior since the identification of HIV as the cause of AIDS. Most of what is known about risk behavior and strategies to change risk behavior are based on studies with homosexual men (Becker & Joseph, 1988; Joseph et al., 1987; Stall, Coates, & Hoff, 1988). It has been long realized that needle sharing is the primary source of infection among heterosexual persons (Chaison, Moss, Onishi, Osmond, & Carlson, 1987). It has been only in the past few years that the need to understand risk behavior associated with heterosexual sex also has been recognized.

Efforts to change sexual risk behavior and increase condom use have been successful in samples of homosexual men. These efforts have included eroticizing condom use in order to promote its use as an enhancement of the sexual interaction (Catania, Gibson, Chitwood, & Coates, 1991) and using peer group leaders to help change group norms to regular use of condoms (Kelly, St. Lawrence, Betts, Brasfield, & Hood, 1990). More recent research, however, has been less encouraging. Young homosexual men are increasingly engaging in high-risk behavior (Ekstrand & Coates, 1990; McKusick, Coates, Morin, Pollack, & Hoff, 1990; Stern, 1990). There is also evidence that condom use is decreasing among homosexual men who previously had been successful in changing their behavior (Joseph, Montgomery, Emmons, Kirscht et al., 1987; McCusker, Zapka, Stoddard, & Mayer, 1989; McKusick, Horstman, & Coates, 1985; Stall, Coates, & Hoff, 1988).

Even without these setbacks, it is unrealistic to assume that the lessons learned from research within one social context (e.g., homosexual men) can be directly applied to a totally different social context (e.g., heterosexual people; Aggleton, O'Reilly, Slutkin, & Davies, 1994). There are important differences between homosexual and heterosexual populations that need to be considered when developing strategies to change heterosexual risk behavior. First is the difference in self-perception of risk: Gay men have recognized from early in the AIDS epidemic that certain sexual acts (e.g., unprotected anal intercourse) put them at increased risk of infection. Heterosexual individuals, however, have been slow to recognize their risk of infection through their sexual activity and, therefore, have been slow to recognize the need for protective behaviors. A second major difference between the two populations is the role that birth control plays in protective behavior. Although fear of pregnancy is not an issue for gay men, it is a primary concern for both heterosexual men and women. When women first become sexually active, condoms provide both birth control and protection against the spread of disease. It is common, however, for women to start using birth control pills when they become increasingly sexually active. They then lose the protection from sexually transmitted diseases that condom use provides.

An additional concern in slowing the continuing spread of HIV infection is the decreasing age at which people are becoming infected. In the early 1980s, the median age was over 30 years old; by 1991, the median age was 25 years. In the period from 1987 to 1991, one of every four newly infected individuals was younger than 22 years (Rosenberg, Biggar, & Goedert, 1994). This fact, along with the awareness that risky sexual behavior is putting the larger heterosexual population at risk, makes college samples important to study.

In a study of a heterosexual sample of college students, Baldwin and Baldwin (1988) investigated the predictors of three measures of sexual risk behavior. The authors reported that age at first intercourse was positively related to frequency of condom use and negatively related to the number of sexual partners in the past 3 months. In other words, the younger the age at which people become sexually active, the less likely they are to use condoms regularly and the more likely they are to have a greater number of sexual partners. Baldwin and Baldwin also reported the following paradoxes. First, people who considered themselves to be at higher risk of contracting AIDS had had a larger number of sexual partners in the preceding 3 months than did people who felt they were at lower risk of infection. Second, people who worried more about contracting AIDS engaged in casual sex more often than those people who were less worried. The authors interpreted these two findings as indicating that the high-risk people knew they were at risk and worried about it, but continued to engage in ·their high-risk behavior.

A questionnaire study of college students' knowledge, beliefs, and behaviors was reported by DiClemente, Forrest, and Mickler (1990). Data from a sample of 1,127 students from 12 different colleges and universities were analyzed. The findings indicated that, in general, these college students were knowledgeable about HIV transmission and AIDS and were sexually active (87%). The study confirmed what other studies have found: There was no association between AIDS knowledge and HIV preventive behavior change. Of great concern to DiClemente et al. was the fact that only 8% of the respondents reported using condoms consistently, and 37% reported never using condoms. The study also revealed that although many students had decreased their risk behaviors, the majority had not and a small percentage had actually increased sexual risk behavior.

Keller (1993) was interested in the reasons young adults gave for not using condoms. In a questionnaire study of 272 young adult college students, respondents completed a questionnaire that provided data about AIDS knowledge and beliefs, difficulties in using condoms, situational and social factors associated with unprotected sexual intercourse, and reasons for unprotected intercourse. A majority (62%) of the respondents reported having had sex at least once without a condom. Although this occurred most often with a partner characterized as a boyfriend or girlfriend (61%), Keller was troubled that unprotected sexual intercourse so often occurred with a relatively casual partner (e.g., "person just met or didn't know well," "person met at a party"). The reasons frequently given for failing to use a condom included intercourse occurred in a long-term relationship; respondents knew the sexual history of the partner; respondents just knew it was safe, or assumed their partner did not have the AIDS virus; and sexual intercourse occurred spontaneously, it was unplanned, or the person just got carried away.

Gerkovich (1995; Gerkovich & Bishop, 1993) has reported two studies of college students. In both studies (*Ns* = 371 and 521, respectively), respondents completed a questionnaire that included items about sexual history and current sexual behavior, knowledge about HIV transmission and AIDS, and a measure of the reversal theory concept of playfulness, spontaneity, and arousal-seeking (paratelic dominance; Cook & Gerkovich, 1993). Both samples had a high level of knowledge, and the majority of respondents were sexually experienced (73% and 71%). The samples were also similar in the frequency of condom use they reported; condoms were consistently used by only 28% in Study 1 and 24% in Study 2. Both of these samples provided data confirming the role of birth control in decisions about condom use with heterosexual individuals. When asked to give reasons for using condoms, men and women in both samples most often gave birth control as the reason, with disease prevention as a secondary reason. When asked for reasons that condoms were not used, both samples included "other forms of birth control were being used" as a major reason. Both studies also documented the role of gender in deciding about condom use. Although the majority of both men and women reported making a joint decision with their partner about condom use, men were much more likely than women to report making the decision by themselves. This finding is not surprising as men are the ones who actually wear condoms. It does emphasize the fact, however, that gender needs to be considered when trying to predict condom use; women must not only make their own decisions, but also negotiate with their male partner. Both studies found that people who were sexually experienced were more arousal-seeking than those who were inexperienced. The second study also found that playfulness and arousal-seeking were related to increased alcohol consumption, which is known to be a risk factor for impaired decision making.

Much of the research on sexual risk behavior has been atheoretical. Theories that have been proposed as being applicable to understanding sexual risk-taking behavior, however, include the health belief model (Kirscht & Joseph, 1989) and the theory of reasoned action (Fishbein & Middlestadt, 1989). The health belief model (i.e., Becker, 1974; Rosenstock, 1974) focuses on behavior that is under an individual's control and is primarily concerned with conscious decisions. The theory of reasoned action (Ajzen & Fishbein, 1980; Fishbein, 1967, 1980) is a general model of behavior that also addresses behaviors that are under volitional control. It focuses on rational thought processes. Joseph and colleagues (Emmons et al., 1986; Joseph, Montgomery, Emmons, Kessler et al., 1987) have reported studies of the relationship between the variables defined by these models and change in AIDS-related behavior among homosexual men. They reported that AIDS knowledge, perceived risk of AIDS, and perceived efficacy of risk behavior change were consistent multivariate predictors of measures reflecting risk behavior change. In a prospective study, they found that perceived social norms (similar to the subjective norms defined in the theory of reasoned action) were a relatively consistent predictor of risk behavior change. Zimmerman and Olson (1994) reported a study in which they tried to predict current sexual risk behavior and change in risk behavior by heterosexual individuals using the health belief model, the theory of reasoned action, and the self-regulatory model of Leventhal and colleagues (e.g., Leventhal, Safer, & Panagis, 1983). In this study, they found that selected variables from all three models explained an additional 8% of the variance in risk behavior change beyond the 10% explained by control variables (e.g., gender, age, race). In terms of current risk behavior, an additional 11% of the variance beyond the 28% explained by the control variables was explained by model variables. The authors concluded that the explanatory power of the models was modest, explaining less of the total variance than control variables such as gender and age. They agreed with other researchers that situational and social context variables need to be incorporated. Cleary (1987) noted that part of the difficulty in modeling preventive health behavior is that the consequences are often delayed and probabilistic. He criticized the application of models developed to address illness behavior and proposed that researchers must move beyond these traditional models and try to get a better understanding of the factors that affect people's assessment of their own risk. Cleary (p. 129) proposed that it is "necessary to recognize that people constantly act without conscious consideration of the consequences of their actions and sometimes act irrationally."

From the research summarized above, it is clear that there is much yet to do if sexual risk-taking behavior among heterosexual individuals is to be understood and changed. More research needs to be done with heterosexual samples, because, as already noted, this group has the fastest increase in rate of new HIV infection. The development and testing of models needs to incorporate findings concerning gender differences as well as the role of birth control options. More needs to be known about how people interpret information about risk and what the factors that influence their evaluation of their own risk are. Models also need to take into account social and situational factors as well as cognitive factors. What follows is a discussion of concepts from reversal theory that are related to sexual risk-taking behavior.

RELEVANT REVERSAL THEORY CONSTRUCTS

The clear relevance of reversal theory to understanding sexual risk behavior is due to two factors: its emphasis on subjective experience (e.g., cognition and affect) rather than behavioral processes alone and its recognition that humans behave in paradoxical ways and are inherently inconsistent. Several constructs from reversal theory can be readily applied to understanding sexual risk-taking behavior. Examples of their relevance were obtained in a pilot study of an interview protocol to obtain information about the situations in which condoms were and were not used (Gerkovich, 1995). In this pilot study, 10 students (5 men and 5 women) were selected from the sample of college students who had completed the questionnaire study (N = 371) and expressed interest in being contacted for the interview study. Selection criteria used responses to questionnaire items to ensure that students were engaged in risk behavior. Students selected for the pilot interview study reported the following: They were sexually experienced and currently sexually active, used condoms sometimes (11%–90% of the time), had had more than two different partners in the past 6 months, had sex more than twice a month, and reported at least one instance of sex with a casual partner. After informed consent procedures were completed, students were asked to describe the circumstances and their thoughts and feelings for two sexual encounters, one during which a condom was used and one when a condom was not used. Students got credit for participating; involvement in research studies was a requirement in their general psychology class.

For people to adopt risk-reduction behaviors (e.g., condom use), they must recognize the risk and identify themselves to be at risk. People are most often in the arousal-seeking, paratelic metamotivational state when they are engaged in sexual activity (Frey, 1991). In that state, they perceive risk as a means of increasing arousal, and they make choices based on a desire for excitement; therefore, risk may be desirable rather than something to be avoided. Acknowledging, and even allowing, a certain level of risk is a means of increasing the excitement that is experienced. This enhancement of the experience by a certain level of risk was expressed by a 19-year-old woman in an interview where she described a sexual encounter in a park, within sight of her boyfriend's house. She stated, "That was scary for me, being out in the open where we could easily be discovered. It was different enough that it made it exciting."

Another important reversal theory concept is the spontaneous, rather than planning-ahead, character of the paratelic metamotivational state. One of the major reasons students reported that condoms were not used is that they were not available when needed (Gerkovich, 1995; Gerkovich & Bishop, 1993). People are often unwilling to acknowledge in advance that sexual activity may occur; letting sex happen spontaneously is more consistent with preferences in the paratelic state. In addition, they are more involved in what they are currently feeling and experiencing while in the paratelic state; decisions are based on current needs and desires, and people are unlikely to think about the long-term consequences of their failure to use a condom. A 19-year-old woman expressed this in an interview: "I had it in the back of my mind that we should be using a condom, but I got so caught up in what was happening that I just didn't care. I didn't even really think about pregnancy."

A third aspect of the paratelic metamotivational state, feeling playful rather than serious-minded, is also important in understanding why condoms are not used. When people are in the paratelic state and are engaged in sexual activity, they are unlikely to consider the serious consequences of not using a condom. A

19-year-old man expressed this when he described his feelings about failing to use a condom on one occasion: "It wasn't planned, it just kind of happened. And I didn't really care at the time."

The above examples are best understood using the reversal theory construct of phenomenological frames (Apter, 1993). Apter used this term because people "frame" their experience, providing a context for what is experienced. One type of frame is the confidence frame, which is experienced during the arousal-seeking state of mind and allows one to have confidence that no harm will occur. This feeling allows a person to experience danger because he or she is confident that there is also protection from that danger. In the case of sexual risk behavior, the protection is not necessarily in the form of protective actions like condom use. Feelings of protection from danger may also arise because people feel they can trust their partners and believe they know their partners' sexual history. In other cases, another kind of frame known as the safety-zone frame may be relevant while in the arousal-seeking state of mind. This frame allows the person to feel protected because there is no perceived danger at all. This frame may be in effect as a result of a person thinking that only other groups (e.g., homosexual people, people who use drugs) are at risk. The third type of phenomenological frame that is relevant to understanding sexual risk-taking behavior is the encapsulation frame that is experienced as part of the playful, spontaneous aspect of the paratelic state. The encapsulation frame allows persons in the paratelic state to feel that their actions are only important in the present, that there are no long-term consequences of their actions.

Other reversal theory constructs are also important for understanding sexual risk-taking behavior. The influence of being in the conformist metamotivational state during sexual activity can either promote or inhibit condom use. As mentioned earlier, research (Kelly, St. Lawrence, Betts, Brasfield, & Hood, 1990) has shown that campaigns to increase condom use have been successful if they have incorporated an aspect of group conformity, making it the acceptable and expected behavior in the person's peer group. Enlisting the aid of recognized group leaders has also been successful in changing risk behavior. Being in the conformist state, however, can work against adopting protective behavior if the partner is opposed to using condoms. This may be more of a problem for women, who are more likely to need to negotiate with their male partners about whether to use a condom (Gerkovich, 1995; Gerkovich & Bishop, 1993). In an interview about a situation in which a condom was not used, an 18-year-old woman described her male partner as being frustrated and mad at her when she asked him to use a condom.

Sexual relations are usually, but not always, conducted while in the sympathy rather than the mastery metamotivational state. This means that the person's preference is for feelings of caring, liking, or loving. Public education efforts and campaigns to increase condom use have tried to present the argument that you are showing concern and care for both you and your partner by using condoms to protect against disease. This argument may be persuasive, but it does not address the feelings expressed by a 19-year-old man in a interview about an occasion when a condom was not used. When asked about his feelings and thoughts after failing to use a condom, he reported, "I felt a little bit better that she didn't care and that maybe she trusted me. . . .It made me feel like she cared more." For this young man, and others like him, the focus of his feelings is caring for his partner and concern for the relationship, not a long-term, probabilistic concern about disease. The weakness of using "trust in partner" as a reason to fail to use a condom was expressed by a female respondent who provided the following answer to an open-ended question concerning the reasons for why condoms are not used: "It's a monogamous relationship, I hope." Even as she used monogamy as a justification for not using condoms, she acknowledged her doubt.

PROPOSED MODEL OF SEXUAL RISK-TAKING

The information presented above illustrates the complexity of the issue of sexual risk-taking behavior among heterosexual individuals. On the basis of the literature on sexual risk behavior, previous questionnaire and interview research, and a review of reversal theory concepts that are relevant, a model to explain sexual risk-taking behavior by heterosexual persons is proposed here. In this model, shown in Figure 1, the outcome variable to be explained is condom use. The figure presents the latent concepts or factors (labeled circles) that influence condom use and affect behavior, attitudes, and beliefs. These latent concepts include paratelic dominance, perceived risk in the relationship, feelings of personal vulnerability, and mediators of condom use. The variables that measure these latent factors (labeled rectangles) are also detailed in Figure 1 and are discussed in detail below. Arrows connecting the latent concepts, and connecting each latent concept to its set of measurement variables, reflect the direction of influence. The model takes into account situational factors as well as factors related to personality, knowledge, beliefs, and past sexual behavior. A description of the proposed model and the relationships accounted for follows.

The reversal theory concept of paratelic dominance influences all other latent concepts in various ways. Paratelic dominance is measured in terms of playfulness, spontaneity, and arousal-seeking. In comparison to people who score low on paratelic dominance, people who score higher will be more likely to have a higher level of risk in their sexual relationships, feel less vulnerable to risks in general, and perceive more barriers to condom use.

A second important concept in explaining condom use, and one that is influenced by paratelic dominance, is perceived risk in the relationship. Level of perceived risk is measured by behavior (e.g., number of different partners and number of casual partners) as well as by type of sexual relationship. People will be aware of being at increased risk in their sexual relationships when they have a larger number of different partners and casual partners. Paradoxically, they will feel they are at less risk if they are involved in a committed sexual relation-

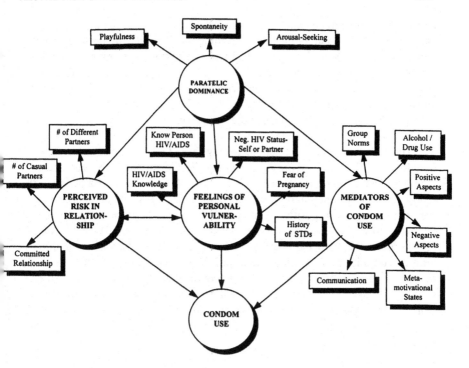

Figure 1 Proposed model of condom use as influenced by paratelic dominance, perceived risk in the relationship, feelings of personal vulnerability, and mediators. Neg. = negative; STDs = sexually transmitted diseases.

ship or feel that they know their partner's previous sexual history and trust them. These last factors (committed relationship and trusting partner) actually decrease the chance that a condom will be used.

Feelings of personal vulnerability will be affected by both level of paratelic dominance and level of perceived risk. Feelings of vulnerability will be increased by such things as knowing someone who is HIV-positive, has AIDS, or has died of AIDS; having accurate information about the risk of HIV transmission; having a history of sexually transmitted diseases; and fear of pregnancy. Decreases in feelings of vulnerability, however, will result from having a negative HIV test result for either self or partner and use of noncondom forms of birth control. People who score high on paratelic dominance will be less likely to take seriously the potential risk their sexual behavior exposes them to and will also be less likely to consider the long-term consequences of their behavior. Level of perceived risk in the relationship will be positively related to level of feelings of vulnerability; as people perceive themselves to be involved in higher risk relationships, they will also feel more vulnerable.

Mediators of condom use can be either positive or negative. Positive mediators include such things as experience with using condoms to increase erotic aspects of the sexual encounter and belief that regular use is the accepted group norm. Negative mediators include such things as inability to communicate desire to use condoms to the partner, resistance of partner to using a condom, not being prepared when condoms are needed, and use of alcohol or drugs. People who score high on paratelic dominance will be more likely to be unprepared when a condom is needed and will be less likely to delay the desires of the moment in order to get a condom. The influences of reversal theory metamotivational states, as described above, will also serve as mediators of condom use.

The model presents the relations among these factors in explaining condom use. Research has already provided support for the relations between some of the measurement variables presented in this model. Baldwin and Baldwin (1988) reported a positive relation between self-perception of risk and number of sexual partners, as well as a positive relation between number of casual partners and the extent to which the person worries about AIDS. Keller (1993) and Gerkovich (1995) found the predicted relation between sexual risk behavior within a long-term or committed relationship. Gerkovich (1995; Gerkovich & Bishop, 1993) also reported support for other relations proposed in the model. Feeling of personal vulnerability was decreased when fear of pregnancy was decreased (e.g., woman was using birth control pills). People who scored higher on paratelic dominance were more likely to use alcohol and were more likely to be sexually experienced.

CONCLUSION

Clearly, this is a very complex model, and much needs to be done to test its validity. Given the issue of gender differences, the model needs to be tested for men as well as for women. It has yet to be determined what relations in the proposed model would differ between men and women. Gerkovich (1995) found that men were more likely to report having sex with a casual partner and consuming alcohol before having sex and were less likely to report speaking to their partners about AIDS. The proposed model is an attempt to address some of the weaknesses in previous model tests. It incorporates reversal theory constructs that are clearly relevant to sexual risk-taking behavior, as well as allowing for the integration of cognitive, emotional, situational, and personality factors.

REFERENCES

Aggleton, P., O'Reilly, K., Slutkin, G., & Davies, P. (1994, July 15). Risking everything? Risk behavior, behavior change, and AIDS. *Science*, 265, 341–345.

Ajzen, I., & Fishbein, M. (1980). *Understanding attitudes and predicting social behavior.* Englewood Cliffs, NJ: Prentice-Hall.

Apter, M. J. (1993). Phenomenological frames and the paradoxes of experience. In J. H. Kerr, S. Murgatroyd, & M. J. Apter (Eds.), *Advances in reversal theory* (pp. 27–39). Amsterdam: Swets & Zeitlinger.

Baldwin, J. D., & Baldwin, J. I. (1988). Factors affecting AIDS-related sexual risk-taking behavior among college students. *Journal of Sex Research, 25,* 181–196.

Becker, M. H. (Ed.). (1974). *The health belief model and personal health behavior.* Thorofare, NJ: Slack.

Becker, M. H., & Joseph, J. G. (1988). AIDS and behavioral change to reduce risk: A review. *American Journal of Public Health, 78,* 394–410.

Catania, J. A., Gibson, D. R., Chitwood, D. D., & Coates, T. J. (1991). Methodological problems in AIDS behavioral research: Influences on measurement error and participant bias in studies of sexual behavior. *Psychological Bulletin, 108,* 339–362.

Chaisson, R. E., Moss, A. R., Onishi, R., Osmond, D., & Carlson, J. R. (1987). Human immunodeficiency virus infection in heterosexual intravenous drug users in San Francisco. *American Journal of Public Health, 77,* 169–172.

Cleary, P. D. (1987). Why people take precautions against health risks. In N. D. Weinstein (Ed.), *Taking care: Understanding and encouraging self-protective behavior* (pp. 119–149). New York: Cambridge University Press.

Cook, M. R., & Gerkovich, M. M. (1993). The development of a Paratelic Dominance Scale. In J. H. Kerr, S. Murgatroyd, & M. J. Apter (Eds.), *Advances in reversal theory* (pp. 177–188). Amsterdam: Swets & Zeitlinger.

DiClemente, R. J., Forrest, K. A., & Mickler, S. (1990). College students' knowledge and attitudes about AIDS and changes in HIV-preventive behaviors. *AIDS Education & Prevention, 2,* 201–212.

Ekstrand, M. L., & Coates, T. J. (1990). Maintenance of safer sexual behaviors and predictors of risky sex: The San Francisco men's health study. *American Journal of Public Health, 80,* 973–977.

Emmons, C. A., Joseph, J. G., Kessler, R. C., Wortman, C. B., Montgomery, S. B., & Ostrow, D. G. (1986). Psychosocial predictors of reported behavior change in homosexual men at risk for AIDS. *Health Education Quarterly, 13,* 341–347.

Fishbein, M. (1967). Attitude and the prediction of behavior. In M. Fishbein (Ed.), *Readings in attitude theory and measurement* (pp. 477–492). New York: Wiley.

Fishbein, M. (1980). A theory of reasoned action: Some applications and implications. In H. E. Howe & M. M. Page (Eds.), *Nebraska Symposium on Motivation, 1979* (pp. 65–116). Lincoln: University of Nebraska Press.

Fishbein, M., & Middlestadt, S. E. (1989). Using the theory of reasoned action as a framework for understanding and changing AIDS-related behaviors. In V. M. Mays, G. W. Albee, & S. F. Schneider (Eds.), *Primary prevention of AIDS: Psychological approaches* (pp. 93–110). Newbury Park, CA: Sage.

Frey, K. P. (1991). Sexual behaviour as adult play. In J. H. Kerr & M. J. Apter (Eds.), *Adult play: A reversal theory approach* (pp. 55–69). Amsterdam: Swets & Zeitlinger.

Gerkovich, M. M. (1995, July). *The role of reversal theory in explaining sexual risk taking by college students.* Paper presented at the Seventh International Conference on Reversal Theory, Melbourne, Victoria, Australia.

Gerkovich, M. M., & Bishop, M. M. (1993, June). *Evidence of reversal theory's relevance to sexual risk taking.* Paper presented at the Sixth International Conference on Reversal Theory, Loftus, Norway.

Joseph, J. G., Montgomery, S. B., Emmons, C. A., Kessler, R. C., Ostrow, D. G., Wortman, C. B., O'Brien, K., Eller, M., & Eshelman, S. (1987). Magnitude and determinants of behavioral risk reduction: Longitudinal analysis of a cohort at risk of AIDS. *Psychology and Health, 1,* 73–95.

Joseph, J. G., Montgomery, S. B., Emmons, C. A., Kirscht, J. P., Kessler, R. C., Ostrow, D. G., Wortman, C. B., & O'Brien, K. (1987). Perceived risk of AIDS: Assessing the behavioral and psychosocial consequences in a cohort of gay men. *Journal of Applied Social Psychology, 17,* 231–250.

Keller, M. L. (1993). Why don't young adults protect themselves against sexual transmission of HIV? Possible answers to a complex question. *AIDS Education & Prevention, 5,* 220–233.

Kelly, J. A., St. Lawrence, J. S., Betts, R. A., Brasfield, T. L., & Hood, H. V. (1990). A skills-training groups intervention model to assist persons in reducing risk behaviors for HIV infection. *AIDS Education & Prevention, 2,* 24–35.

Kirscht, J. P., & Joseph, J. G. (1989). The health belief model: Some implications for behavior change, with reference to homosexual males. In V. M. Mays, G. W. Albee, & S. F. Schneider (Eds.), *Primary prevention of AIDS: Psychological approaches* (pp. 111–127). Newbury Park, CA: Sage.

Leventhal, H., Safer, M. A., & Panagis, D. M. (1983). The impact of communications on the self-regulation of health beliefs, decisions, and behaviors. *Health Education Quarterly, 10/11,* 3–30.

McCusker, J., Zapka, J. G., Stoddard, A. M., & Mayer, K. H. (1989). Responses to the AIDS epidemic among homosexually active men: Factors associated with preventive behavior. *Patient Education and Counselling, 13,* 15–30.

McKusick, L., Coates, T. J., Morin, S. F., Pollack, L., & Hoff, C. (1990). Longitudinal predictors of reductions in unprotected anal intercourse among gay men in San Francisco: The AIDS behavioral research project. *American Journal of Public Health, 80,* 978–983.

McKusick, L., Horstman, W., & Coates, T. J. (1985). AIDS and sexual behavior reported by gay men in San Francisco. *American Journal of Public Health, 75,* 493–496.

Rosenberg, P. S., Biggar, R. J., & Goedert, J. J. (1994). Declining age at HIV infection in the United States. *New England Journal of Medicine, 330,* 789–790.

Rosenstock, I. M. (1974). Historical origins of the health belief model. *Health Education Monographs, 2,* 328–335.

Stall, R. D., Coates, T. J., & Hoff, C. (1988). Behavioral risk reduction for HIV infection among gay and bisexual men. *American Psychologist, 43,* 878–885.

Stern, M. J. (1990, April). *Reasons for having sex as predictors of condom use.* Paper presented at the Eleventh Scientific Sessions of the Society of Behavioral Medicine, Chicago, IL.

Zimmerman, R. S., & Olson, K. (1994). AIDS-related risk behavior and behavior change in a sexually active, heterosexual sample: A test of three models of prevention. *AIDS Education & Prevention, 6,* 189–205.

V

HEALTH-PROMOTING BEHAVIOR

12

Motives for Donating Blood

Michael J. Apter and Naomi Spirn

A questionnaire generated from within the framework of reversal theory was administered to 217 volunteers at a student blood drive, together with a before-and-after emotion checklist. The questionnaire included questions about motives for giving blood, couched in terms of the eight basic metamotives postulated in reversal theory (i.e., the motives underlying each of the eight metamotivational states). Results showed that, not surprisingly, the primary reason for giving blood was that of alloic sympathy (caring for others). Other metamotives were, however, also implicated for many volunteers, both in terms of responses to the questionnaire and to the checklist. These included especially the telic motive of doing things that are meaningful and important, the conformist motive of doing the moral thing, and the mastery motive of overcoming one's own fears. All eight metamotives, in fact, could be discerned in the responses of at least some participants. An implication is that appeals for donors should rely on more than the motive of altruism.

Finding ways to encourage people to donate blood is a perennial problem for medical services, and for the community at large. Clearly, any improvement in understanding what all the different motives are of those people who do give blood without monetary reward would be helpful in improving the recruitment of new donors or in encouraging those who have already given blood to continue to do so on a regular basis.

The central problem is this: Why do people give blood? In commonsense

The authors' thanks are due to the following individuals, and the organizations they represent, for giving us permission to collect data during blood drives: John Alli of the Blood Preservation Laboratory, Cook County Hospital, Chicago, Illinois; Jill R. Danielson of the United Blood Services, Chicago Center, Chicago, Illinois; and Karie Hakanson of the Student Blood Services, Northwestern University, Evanston, Illinois. Our thanks are also due to Andrea Lerner and Mary Beth Leisen for their help in data collection.

145

terms, the main motive is obviously the altruistic one of helping others, and this commonsense idea has been generally supported in the research literature (e.g., see review by Boe & Ponder, 1981). The importance of developing the altruistic identity of being a blood giver has also been emphasized in the important research of Piliavin and her group (see Piliavin 1989, 1992; Piliavin & Callero, 1991). If other motives can also be identified, however, and these are motives that can be used to appeal to potential donors or satisfied in such a way as to provide fulfillment to more regular donors, then this would clearly be helpful to know. Certainly other motives have been documented from time to time, for example, sensation-seeking (Farnill & Ball, 1982). Altruistic motives have not always been found to be the most important factor (Condie, Warner, & Gillman, 1976). Yet, researchers in this field have tended to focus on a rather narrow band of related motives, especially the need to help others, the need to improve self-esteem, and the need to conform to social pressures that arise from community needs (see review in Piliavin & Callero, 1991). The result is that it is possible that other motives that may enter into the decision to give blood, or to continue to give blood, may have been overlooked.

This chapter documents donor motivation in a way that is sensitive to a variety of possible motives over and above those of altruism. In other words, it involves what has been called *functional analysis,* defined as an analysis that is "concerned with the reasons and purposes that underlie and generate psychological phenomena" (Clary & Snyder, 1991, p. 123). Piliavin and Callero (1991) have called for more theoretically based research on blood donation, and reversal theory provides a theoretical framework that allowed the present authors to approach this area in a systematic way.

By asking participants about all their metamotives in relation to their action of giving blood, it was possible to carry out a form of functional analysis of such an action that might be referred to more specifically as metamotivational analysis. By *metamotive* here is meant a motive that underlies a metamotivational state (e.g., the motive to have fun in the paratelic state and the motive to break free of rules in the negativistic state). To implement this form of analysis, a questionnaire was devised in which the key item provided participants with a set of motivational statements that they could endorse as descriptors of their own motivation or motivations for donating blood. Each metamotive was represented by a single statement of this kind, written in a way to make it potentially relevant to blood donation. In developing the questionnaire, all these statements were put in such as way as to be, in principle, desirable. Participants were also given the option of contributing their own statements if they could find no suitable match with any of those given in the list provided.

An emotion checklist was also provided both before and after donation for participants to indicate the particular emotions they were experiencing at each of these times. The emotion checklist was not an arbitrary collection of emotions but was derived from those identified in reversal theory as being basic (Apter 1989; see also Chapter 1, specifically Figure 1). Similar sets of emotion nouns have been used in other reversal theory research, notably that involving the Tension and Effort Stress Inventory (Svebak, 1993; see also Chapter 5).

The principal aim of the research was first to ask donors directly about their motives for donating blood and second to examine the before-to-after changes of emotion in donors, as an additional guide to their underlying motives. In this case, reversal theory did not provide specific hypotheses for testing but rather acted as a framework for essentially descriptive and exploratory research.

RESEARCH METHOD: BLOOD COLLECTION

Participants

Participants were students at Northwestern University in Illinois who volunteered to donate their blood during two separate blood drives that took place on the Evanston campus of the university, under the auspices of the Student Blood Service. Technical blood collection services for the first blood drive were provided by United Blood Services; for the second, by Cook County Hospital. Participation in the study among the donors was voluntary; only a few of those approached declined to participate. Participants from the first drive were excluded from acting as participants in the second drive. The number of participants who participated from the first drive was 164 (90 women, 74 men); from the second drive, 53 (22 women, 31 men). Data from both drives was combined for purposes of data analysis to produce a population of 217.

Materials

The materials consisted of the following two questionnaires.

The Blood Donation Questionnaire

This questionnaire asked the following questions:

1 How often have you given blood before?
2 When was the last time?
3 Do you see this as a regular part of your life? YES/NO
4 Do you encourage others to give blood, or do you believe that it is up to each individual to make up their own minds? (Please check one below:)
     Encourage others
     Up to each individual
5 Do you intend to give blood again?
6 Why do you donate blood? Please check all of the statements below that you feel apply to you in your decision to give blood.
   a I like to do things that are meaningful and important.
   b I like to have intense experiences.
   c I feel it is the right and moral thing to do.

---

d I think we need to show up those who are too selfish to help others.
e I want to master my own fears and weaknesses.
f I think that we need to put the needs of society before our own.
g I feel that others appreciate me for what I do.
h I want to help other individuals in need.
i Other (please specify):
7 Which of the feelings or motives described above is the one that is the most important of all? Please write the letter corresponding to it here:
8 What do you think is the main reason why some people refuse to give blood? (Please check those below that you think apply.)
a Afraid (e.g., of pain or of contracting AIDS)
b Shortsightedness
c Friends and acquaintances do not do it
d Refusal to be pressured into things
e Do not wish to lose control
f Enough other people do it
g Selfishness
h Feel that they choose to give in other ways
i Other (please specify):
9 Of the reasons listed above for not giving blood, which do you feel is the single most important one for most people? Please write the letter corresponding to the reason here:

Emotion Checklist
The Emotion Checklist came in a "before" and an "after" version. The before version asked donors to check all those emotions that they were experiencing while waiting to give blood and the after version asked them to check all those emotions that they were experiencing after having given blood. The list of emotions was the same in each case and consisted of the following: anxiety, relaxation, excitement, boredom, anger, provocativeness, virtue, guilt, resentment, gratitude, triumph, humiliation, modesty, and shame. Respondents were also asked to write in any emotions not listed that they might be experiencing at the time in question.

Procedure

Potential participants were approached at the blood donor registration desk. If they agreed to participate in the study, they were asked to read and sign a consent form and to complete the *before* emotion checklist. The *after* emotion checklist, and the main questionnaire, were administered to the consenting participants during the rest period after their blood had been drawn. (During the rest period, participants sit quietly and are given something to eat and drink.) Questionnaires could be filled in anonymously, or names could be given.

MOTIVATION AND EMOTION

Participant Characteristics

- Eighty-five percent of the male participants and 75% of the female participants had given blood before, the modal number of times for both men and women being once.
- The modal number of months since previous donations among participants who had donated before was 2 months for both men and women.
- Sixty-six percent of the men and 77% of the women saw blood donation as a regular part of their lives.
- Sixty percent of the men and 63% of the women reported that they encouraged others to give blood.
- Eighty-six percent of the men and 94% of the women reported that they intended to give blood again.

Motives for Donating Blood

The reasons people donate blood are summarized in Figure 1 for men and women separately. This figure shows the percentage of respondents who checked each motive (rounded out to the nearest percentage point). Percentages have been used because the sample size is different for men and women, making

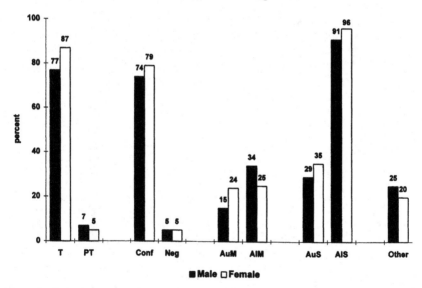

Figure 1 Percentage of participants endorsing each metamotive for their blood donation, where any number of such metamotives could be endorsed by each participant. T = telic, PT = paratelic, Conf = conformist, Neg = negativistic, AuM = autic mastery, AIM = alloic mastery, AusS = autic sympathy, AIS = alloic sympathy.

absolute comparisons between the sexes less immediately meaningful to visual inspection. For further explanation, refer to Item 6 of the Blood Donation Questionnaire. The responses to this item related to the metamotivational states shown in the figure in the following way: Telic corresponded to Response a on Item 6 of the Blood Donation Questionnaire ("I like to do things that are meaningful and important"); paratelic to Response b of the questionnaire; conformist to Response c; negativistic to Response d; autic mastery to Response e; alloic mastery to Response f; autic sympathy to Response g; and alloic sympathy to Response h.

An alternative way of measuring the frequency of different motives is for each participant to choose the single most important motive for him or her. The results of this measure of popularity from Item 7 of the Blood Donation Questionnaire, which calls for this kind of choice, are summarized in Figure 2, again for men and women separately. Again, to make visual inspection easier, percentages have been used in the histogram and rounded out to the nearest percentage point. (Five participants failed to answer this question [1 man and 4 women], and so the percentages are based on a lower sample size for each sex.) Because each participant is equally represented in the data from Item 7, with a single choice, it is possible to perform a chi-square test on the total distribution. This confirms what is obvious from the pattern shown in the histogram: The null hypothesis is rejected for both men and women at a level well beyond $p <$

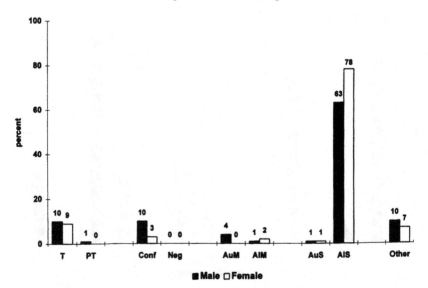

Figure 2 Percentage of participants endorsing each metamotive for their blood donation, where only the single most important motive could be endorsed by each participant. T = telic, PT = paratelic, Conf = conformist, Neg = negativistic, AuM = autic mastery, AlM = alloic mastery, AusS = autic sympathy, AlS = alloic sympathy.

.001. χ^2 for men (8, N = 104) was 301.24, and for women (8, N = 108) it was 494.82. Also, the distribution for men is not significantly different from that for women, χ^2(8, N = 212) = 11.00, p > .05.

Reasons for Not Giving Blood

The reasons that donors believed that other people might have for refusing to give blood (Item 8 of the Blood Donation Questionnaire) are summarized in Figure 3. As explained earlier when discussing Figure 1 and Item 6 of the Blood Donation Questionnaire, absolute numbers have been converted to percentages to allow comparison between the sexes.

Figure 4 shows the endorsement frequency of different responses where the respondent has to make a choice of one motive only (Item 9 of the Blood Donation Questionnaire). Again, the absolute numbers have been converted to percentages. (Three male participants failed to respond to this item, meaning that the percentages are based here on a sample size of 102; 1 female participant failed to respond, meaning that the percentages are based here on a sample size of 111.) Using chi-square, the null hypothesis was rejected for both men and women; men, χ^2(8, N = 102) = 316.5, p < .001; women, χ^2(8, N = 111) = 415.29, p < .001. As for motives for donating blood, there was no significant difference between men and women, χ^2(8, N = 213) = 5.50, p > .05.

All Motives For Not Donating Blood

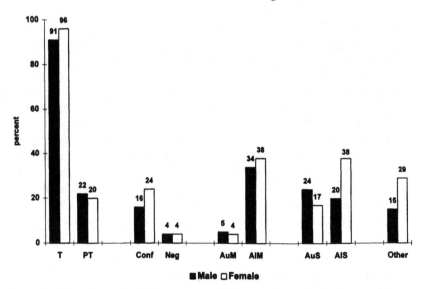

Figure 3 Percentage of participants endorsing each metamotive as a reason for not giving blood, where any number of such metamotives could be endorsed by each participant. T = telic, PT = paratelic, Conf = conformist, Neg = negativistic, AuM = autic mastery, AIM = alloic mastery, AusS = autic sympathy, AIS = alloic sympathy.

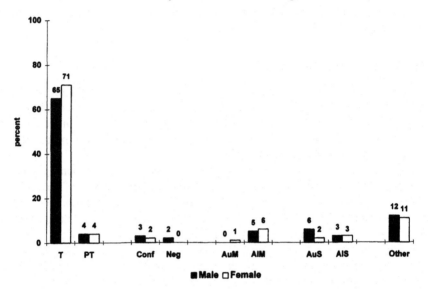

Figure 4 Percentage of participants endorsing each metamotive as a reason for not giving blood, where only the single most important motive could be endorsed by each participant. T = telic, PT = paratelic, Conf = conformist, Neg = negativistic, AuM = autic mastery, AIM = alloic mastery, AusS = autic sympathy, AIS = alloic sympathy.

Emotion Change

Figure 5 shows the before and after frequencies for the emotions identified in the emotion checklist. Because there were no clear sex differences, these were summed across both sexes. It will be noticed that those emotions displaying the most marked change were anxiety, relaxation, boredom, excitement, virtue, and triumph. Using the McNemar test for the significance of changes, all of these emotions displayed change at a significant level ($p < .001$ for anxiety, excitement, boredom, and triumph; $p < .01$ for virtue; and $p < .05$ for relaxation).

There were a small number of write-in emotions, which were in the main simply different hedonic tone words like *gladness* and *happiness*. The one exception was *relief*, which was written in by 1 participant in the before condition and 20 in the after condition. This would appear to be essentially a synonym for *relaxation* and amplifies further the before-and-after difference in relation to the latter emotion.

EXAMINATION OF THE QUESTIONNAIRE

The central items in the questionnaire are Items 6 and 7, asking volunteers to indicate their reasons for donating blood. If one look at Figures 1 and 2, one sees that the "help others" response category is the one that shows the most

Before-and-After Emotions

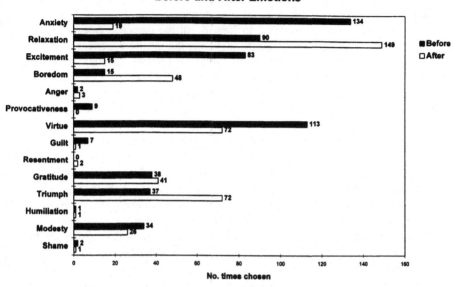

Figure 5 Number of times each emotion was endorsed as a self-descriptor, over all participants (N = 217), before and after donating blood.

strongly, both in the unrestricted case where participants may check as many categories as they wish (Figure 1) and in the restricted case where participants may choose a single category (Figure 2). In reversal theory terms, this is the response category that represents alloic sympathy, essentially the prosocial or altruistic motive. This result is of course not surprising and is consistent with previous research, as noted in the introduction to this chapter. It is interesting, though, that the "desire to be appreciated" response (autic sympathy) was checked considerably less often, implying that the altruism is, if respondents are being truthful, a genuine desire to help others rather than, as some cynics might have asserted, no more than a desperate attempt to find a way to be liked.

Of even more interest is the strong showing of the first response category, which is worded in the questionnaire "I like to do things that are meaningful and important." In reversal theory terms, this is the telic motive. It means that participants hope, to some degree, to give meaning and significance to their lives through the action of donating blood. If one compare Figures 1 and 2, one can conclude that, although this is not most donors' primary motive, it is a secondary motive for a large majority.

Not far behind in response popularity in Figure 2 comes the moral motive (in reversal theory terms, a type of conformist response) "I feel it is the right and moral thing to do." Again, a large majority of participants checked this response (although from Figure 2 one can see that it is the primary motive in only a small number of cases). The importance of this motive is consistent with the finding of Chliaoutakis, Trakas, Socrataki, and Lemonidou (1994) that feelings of guilt predispose people to become donors.

It is notable that in response to Item 6, all the response categories were checked by at least some participants, including the intense experience category (a form of paratelic sensation-seeking) and the hostile (negativistic) "I think we need to show up those who are too selfish to help others." Reversal theory asserts that human actions are frequently determined by multiple motives, even in the same person, and this would certainly appear to be borne out by the present data in relation to the act of giving blood. In trying to persuade people to behave in certain ways, such as to become donors, it is therefore always well to bear this in mind.

As reported above, no real sex differences emerged, the pattern of motive endorsement being remarkably similar across both sexes for both the unrestricted and restricted response items (Items 6 and 7, respectively). This implies that appeals to men and women can be couched essentially in the same terms.

How far did the options, listed as "a–h" in Item 6 actually capture the full range of motives? This can be assessed by looking at the "other" option in this item. In fact, the write-in responses here fell into four classes: (a) synonymous phrases, that is, different ways of stating reasons already given in the list (e.g., "obligated by religion," which is essentially the same as doing "the right and moral thing" and is in any case a similarly conformist response); (b) simple tautological statements like "it makes me feel good"; (c) autobiographical or circumstantial reasons, such "a friend of mine was recently hospitalized"; and (d) genuinely unexpected reasons, like "to meet women" and "for the free food." On the whole, then, the prewritten reasons given in the list worked as well as could have been expected, with few written-in responses that could not be easily assimilated to the set of metamotives postulated by reversal theory, or the particular versions of them suggested in the list.

Items 8 and 9 of the questionnaire asked about reasons for not giving blood. Although couched in terms of other people's reasons for refusing, the aim of these two items was really to uncover what kinds of conflicts there might have been in volunteers' own decisions. Overwhelmingly here the telic reason—that of fear—was the one that was most endorsed. Interestingly, then, the telic state, in different aspects (serious significance-seeking vs. the desire to avoid arousal), was strongly implicated in the decision both to give and not to give blood. As before, responses written in the *other* category could be largely assimilated to the reasons offered in the prewritten list. The main exception was that of medical reasons, which generally meant having blood that was unsuitable for some medical reason.

As far as changes in emotions are concerned, from before to after donating blood, it has already been noted that six emotions changed in frequency to a significant extent. Looking at this more closely, it is notable that the two high-arousal emotions (anxiety and excitement) both showed a marked drop and the two low-arousal emotions (relaxation and boredom), taken together, showed an increase. This shows that one strong, and not surprising, before-to-after change is that of a lowering of arousal, whatever the metamotivational states involved. It is more surprising that some participants chose the paratelic descriptors (excitement and boredom) to describe their state before donation, implying that for some the situation was not a serious one for them. However, the majority of participants chose telic descriptors (anxiety and relaxation), both before and after (392 telic choices, summing across before and after, against 175 paratelic choices), and this is consistent with the overall preponderance of telic over paratelic choices in answer to Item 6 on the questionnaire. Furthermore, the most frequently chosen response before donation was anxiety, and the most frequent response afterward was relaxation; this implies that for the majority of participants, the telic state was operative throughout, with no reversal taking place. This further implies that the situation was not seen by these telic-state volunteers as one of threat, which on removal would be likely to induce the paratelic state (see Chapter 10), but one of commitment to something unpleasant, whose accomplishment can be enjoyed afterward. In the light of this, perhaps one can make sense of the fact that virtue (an alloic sympathy emotion) decreases as a salient emotion before-to-after, whereas triumph (an autic mastery emotion) increases. That is, it is possible that many volunteers came to the situation in an altruistic sympathy state of mind, but once in the situation saw it as an unpleasant task to be mastered and felt triumphant once they had done so.

CONCLUSION

Although the prosocial motive in this, as in most earlier research, proved itself to be predominant, the study described in this chapter also emphasized the full range of metamotives to be implicated to different degrees (in the same person and across people). As in so much reversal theory research, doubt was cast on the simple idea that a particular action has a particular and unequivocal underlying motive, even in the same person at different times.

Besides the prosocial motive (in reversal theory terms, the alloic sympathy metamotive), telic motivation proved to be particularly important (i.e., the motive of giving oneself a sense of purpose, direction, and meaningfulness). This was apparent not only in the unrestricted choice of reasons for giving blood (Item 6 in the questionnaire), but also in the before-to-after emotion self-descriptions, and in the fact that the majority of participants had given blood before (Item 1) and saw it as a regular part of their lives (Item 3). The importance of the mastery metamotive in some participants (in response to the before-and-after questions) was also notable. In this respect, one volunteer suggested that, at least for some people, there was a kind of "medical rush," similar to the "exercise rush" experienced by many after strenuous physical activity. The other particularly relevant motive was the conformist one of doing the moral thing.

The final conclusion, therefore, must be that in appealing for new donors, and in attempting to retain those who have previously donated blood, it may be advantageous to emphasize the possibility of satisfying a number of basic motives in addition to the motive of altruism.

REFERENCES

Apter, M. J. (1989). *Reversal theory: Motivation, emotion and personality*. London: Routledge.

Boe, G. P., & Ponder, L. D. (1981). Blood donors and non-donors: A review of the research. *American Journal of Medical Technology, 47*, 248–253.

Chliaoutakis, J., Trakas, D. J., Socrataki, F., & Lemonidou, C. (1994). Blood donor behavior in Greece: Implications for health policy. *Social Science and Medicine, 38*, 1461–1467.

Clary, E. G., & Snyder, M. (1991). A functional analysis of altruism and prosocial behavior: The case of volunteerism. In M. Clark (Ed.), *Review of personality and social psychology* (Vol. 12, pp. 119–148). Newbury Park, CA: Sage.

Condie, S. J., Warner, W. K., & Gillman, D. C. (1976). Getting blood from collective turnips: Volunteer donation in mass blood drives. *Journal of Applied Psychology, 61*, 290–294.

Farnill, D., & Ball, I. C. (1982). Sensation-seeking and intention to donate blood. *Psychological Reports, 51*, 126.

Piliavin, J. A. (1989). The development of motives, self-identities and values tied to blood dona-tion: A Polish-American comparison study. In N. Eisenberg, J. Reykowski, & E. Staub (Eds.), *Social and moral values: Individual and societal perspectives* (pp. 253–276). Hillsdale, NJ: Erlbaum.

Piliavin, J. A. (1992). Role identity and organ donation: Some suggestions based on blood dona-tion research. In J. Shanteau & R. J. Harris (Eds.), *Organ donation and transplantation: Psychological and behavioral factors* (pp. 150–158). Washington, DC: American Psychological Association.

Piliavin, J. A., & Callero, P. L. (1991). *Giving blood: The development of an altruistic identity*. Baltimore: Johns Hopkins University Press.

Svebak, S. (1993). The development of the tension and effort stress inventory (TESI). In J. H. Kerr, S. Murgatroyd, & M. J. Apter (Eds.), *Advances in reversal theory* (pp.189–204). Amsterdam: Swets & Zeitlinger.

13

Resisting Urges and Adopting New Behaviors

Kathleen A. O'Connell and Evelyn Brooks

Health promotion experts and clinicians dealing with patients who are chronically ill often recommend changing habits. This chapter takes a reversal theory approach to examining the differences between resisting urges to carry out old habits and adopting new habits. A sample of 242 participants was asked to remember a time when they tried to change a habit. Participants were randomly assigned to one of four recall tasks: (a) a time when they succeeded in resisting an urge to carry out an old habit, (b) a time when they failed in resisting an urge to carry out an old habit, (c) a time when they succeeded in carrying out a new behavior, and (d) a time when they failed at carrying out a new behavior. Participants answered a 46-item questionnaire designed to assess telic–paratelic, arousal-avoidant/arousal-seeking, negativistic–conformist, and various types of mastery–sympathy states they were experiencing after their success or failure. Results indicated that success in the episodes reported by the participants was associated with being in telic and conformist states. Although metamotivational states did not differ between episodes where urges were successfully resisted and episodes where new behaviors were successfully performed, states did differ between episodes in which participants failed to resist urges and episodes in which participants failed to perform new behaviors. Participants who failed to resist urges were more likely to be classified as paratelic and sympathy-gaining than participants who failed to carry out a new behavior. The implications of these findings for long-term behavior change are discussed.

This chapter is based on a paper originally presented at the 7th International Reversal Theory Conference, July 1995, Melbourne, Victoria, Australia. This study was funded by Grant NR03145 to Kathleen A. O'Connell from the National Institute for Nursing Research, National Institutes of Health, U.S. Dept of Health and Human Services. The authors wish to thank Monica Scheibmeir for her help in developing the Autic Mastery–Sympathy State Measure.

Changing health behaviors is the target of many health promotion and illness management efforts. To avoid heart disease, people are counseled to quit smoking, begin an exercise regimen, and consume a diet that is low in saturated fats. Similar recommendations are given to individuals who have diagnosed heart ailments. Much attention has been given to the difficulty of changing such lifestyle behaviors, and studies have shown that relapse is a common outcome (Brownell, Marlatt, Lichtenstein, & Wilson, 1986). Adopting a healthy lifestyle usually requires two types of behavior change: stopping old habits and starting new ones. Little attention has been given to the differences in these two types of behavior change. Nevertheless, it is clear that stopping an old habit is a different process and requires different skills than acquiring a new habit. For instance, stopping an old habit, such as eating high-fat foods, usually requires the individual to resist urges to resume the old habit. When the old habit involves an addictive behavior, like smoking, this urge may be especially problematic. Adopting a new behavior, such as exercise, requires the individual to work the behavior into his or her life. Although resisting urges to do alternative behaviors (e.g., resisting the urge to sleep rather than do morning exercise) may be involved in adopting new behaviors, the urge component is usually not as problematic as it is with stopping old habits. The consequences of specific instances of success or failure at changing habits may also be different for the two types of behavior change. Although people often find it difficult to engage in a new behavior, like exercise, they usually feel positive after an exercise session. Resisting the urge to eat dessert is also difficult. However, succeeding in doing so can result in the short-term negative consequence of feeling that one is deprived of a treat to which one is entitled. Moreover, the uncomfortable urge may persist or reappear, as does the urge for a cigarette during smoking cessation.

Previous work related to this issue has focused on the metamotivational antecedents of succeeding or failing at resisting the urge to smoke cigarettes during a cessation attempt. Participants who succumbed to the urge to smoke were likely to be in paratelic, negativistic, and sympathy states at the time they decided to smoke, whereas participants who resisted were more likely to be in telic, conformist, and mastery states (Cook, Gerkovich, O'Connell, & Potocky, 1995; O'Connell, Cook, Gerkovich, Potocky, & Swan, 1990; O'Connell, Gerkovich, & Cook, 1995; Potocky, Gerkovich, O'Connell, & Cook, 1991). Popkess-Vawter and Wendel (1995) have also applied reversal theory to overeating episodes. They found that normal-weight women tend to overeat in paratelic states, whereas overweight women tend to overeat in telic states. In contrast to the previous studies, which involved the metamotivational states that are antecedent to lapsing or overeating, this study looked at the metamotivational states that are the consequences of succeeding or failing at carrying out health behaviors. This study also includes data on adopting new health behaviors. No prior studies have focused on the metamotivational states that are operative when adopting new health behaviors.

The purpose of this study was to compare the experiences of carrying out new health behaviors with resisting urges to carry out old unhealthy behaviors. Specifically, the metamotivational states experienced as a consequence of succeeding and failing at resisting urges and adopting new behaviors were investigated. The following research questions were addressed.

In terms of the telic–paratelic, negativistic–conformist, and mastery–sympathy metamotivational variables,

1   Which states are associated with success in changing each type of behavior?

2   How does the experience of success at resisting an urge to carry out an established behavior differ from the experience of success at carrying out a new behavior?

3   How does the experience of failure at resisting an urge to carry out an established behavior differ from the experience of failure at carrying out a new behavior?

CHANGING HEALTH BEHAVIORS: METHOD OF THE STUDY

Participants

The sample for the study consisted of 242 students or employees of a large medical center in the central United States. The age of the participants varied from 16 to 59, with a mean age of 29 years. Seventy-three percent of the sample were female; 76% were Caucasian, 10% African American, 8% Asian, 3% Hispanic, and 2% American Indian.

Instrument

The instrument was a 46-item questionnaire containing four subscales: Serious–Playful, Arousal-Avoidant/Arousal-Seeking, Negativistic–Conformist, and Mastery–Sympathy. The items of the subscales were intermixed and presented in random order.

Telic–Paratelic Pair   The telic–paratelic pair was assessed by two subscales: Serious–Playful (four items) and Arousal-Avoidance/Arousal-Seeking (three items). The items had four response alternatives. Thus, the Serious–Playful subscale had a range of 4 to 16 with a midpoint of 10, and the Arousal-Avoidant/Arousal-Seeking subscale had a range of 3 to 12 with a midpoint of 8. The selection of items for these subscales was based on the Somatic State Questionnaire developed by Cook, Gerkovich, Potocky, and O'Connell (1993), with revisions suggested by Calhoun and O'Connell (1995). In this sample, the coefficient alphas were .80 for the Serious–Playful subscale and .59 for the Arousal-Avoidance/Arousal-Seeking subscale. The midpoint of each scale was used as the cutpoint for categorizing participants as either serious or playful and as either arousal-seeking or arousal-avoidant.

Negativistic–Conformist Pair   The negativistic–conformist pair was assessed with the four items of the Negativistic–Conformist subscale of the Somatic State Questionnaire developed by Cook and Gerkovich. Each item had four response options, giving the Negativistic–Conformist subscale a range of 4 to 16 with a midpoint of 10. The midpoint was used to classify each participant as conformist or negativistic. In this sample, the coefficient alpha of the scale was .60.

Mastery–Sympathy Pair   The mastery–sympathy pair was assessed with the Autic Mastery–Sympathy State Measure (AuMSSM) developed by the authors. The mastery–sympathy pair presents a difficult measurement challenge. Because of its conceptual linkage to the autic–alloic pair, it was necessary to assess mastery and sympathy within the context of the autic and alloic pair. In previous work with smoking cessation, it has been found that alloic states occur infrequently in the types of situations we were interested in exploring (O'Connell, Gerkovich, & Cook, 1995). Thus, to decrease the complexity of the task, the authors limited the scale development to autic states. It should be noted that there are two versions of the autic state: autocentric, wherein the participant is interacting with an outside agent, and intra-autic, wherein the participant is interacting with the self (i.e., *I* vs. *me*). The mastery–sympathy pair reverses on the felt toughness dimension (O'Connell & Apter, 1993). In addition, mastery and sympathy states also have been described in terms of the gaining–losing dimension (Apter & Smith, 1985). Both dimensions were considered in the development of items for the AuMSSM.

A review of items used for assessing the telic–paratelic pair and the negativistic–conformist pair revealed that the items are generally neutral with respect to hedonic tone. Thus, the items for the serious–playful measures address whether the participant is playful or serious, not the level of hedonic tone the participant is feeling. A participant could be playful but experiencing either pleasant or unpleasant hedonic tone. After several attempts at developing a mastery–sympathy measure, it was decided that it would be expedient to factor into the assessment whether the participant was experiencing positive or negative hedonic tone with respect to the mastery–sympathy pair. Rather than choosing items that were neutral with respect to hedonic tone, it was found that items representing either losing or gaining on the transactional outcome dimension (e.g., feeling neglected or appreciated on the sympathy side, self-disciplined and undisciplined on the mastery side) and items representing tough and tender on the felt toughness dimension (e.g., affectionate or deprived on the sympathy side, assertive or weak on the mastery side) made more sense to participants and produced more usable scales. Initially, a list of 81 items derived from a lexicon of mastery–sympathy descriptors (O'Connell, 1993) and antonyms and synonyms of these descriptors contained in the thesaurus listings of two word-processing software packages were generated. Pilot testing produced a list of 34 items that were used in a subsequent instrument development study.

To arrive at a smaller set of items to assess mastery–sympathy states, a discriminant function analysis approach was used to select an item set that discriminated between mastery and sympathy states.

Participants were asked to read scenarios describing various types of mastery and sympathy states and to remember the last time they had experienced a similar situation. Then they were asked to respond to the 34-item measure of mastery–sympathy states as they would have during that particular experience. To control for the effects of item order, three different orderings of the items were used. Eight different scenarios were developed, representing different types of autic mastery and autic sympathy states. The following list shows the types of states and a brief description of the scenarios. The scenarios vary in three different ways: (a) whether they depict autocentric or intra-autic versions of the autic states, (b) whether they depict mastery or sympathy states, and (c) whether they depict gaining or losing. The scenarios were reviewed for content validity by Michael Apter and were pilot tested on several groups of participants. Revisions in the scenario descriptions and examples were made on the basis of the pilot test findings.

The Scenarios Used to Develop the Autic Mastery–Sympathy State Measure

1 Autocentric mastery-gaining—I succeeded at mastering something or defeating someone, and I felt good about it.

2 Autocentric mastery-losing—I failed at mastering something or defeating someone, and I felt bad about it.

3 Autocentric sympathy-gaining—I felt liked or loved by someone else, and I felt good about it.

4 Autocentric sympathy-losing—I felt unloved or disliked by someone else, and I felt bad about it.

5 Intra-autic mastery-gaining—I succeeded in getting myself to do something I should do, and I felt pleased about it.

6 Intra-autic mastery-losing—I failed to do something that I think is for my own good, and I felt bad about it.

7 Intra-autic sympathy-gaining—I allowed myself to indulge in something I enjoy, and I felt pleased with myself.

8 Intra-autic sympathy-losing—I did not allow myself to do something I really enjoyed, and I felt cheated.

A sample of 331 participants each responded to two scenarios. Three separate discriminant function analyses were carried out. In the first analysis, a stepwise procedure was used to select, from the 34 items in the data set, the set of items that best discriminated between scenarios depicting losing situations from scenarios depicting gaining situations. A second stepwise discriminant function analysis was carried out to select variables that distinguished mastery-gaining scenarios from sympathy-gaining scenarios. A third stepwise discriminant function analysis was carried out to distinguish mastery-losing scenarios from sympathy-losing scenarios. The variables selected in each analysis appear in the following list. Because this study focused on intra-autic states, which concern mastering oneself or giving sympathy to oneself, two additional items were added to ensure that variables relevant to the intra-autic state were included ("kind to self" to represent sympathy-gaining and "depriving self" to represent sympathy-losing). Because this scale addresses only autic states and not alloic states, losing is always associated with negative hedonic tone and gaining is always associated with positive hedonic tone.

Subscales of the Autic Mastery–Sympathy State Measure

  I Gaining–Losing Scale
- **A** assertive
- **B** appreciated
- **C** kind to self
- **D** *weak
- **E** *depriving self
- **F** *undisciplined
- **G** *not cared about

 II Mastery-Gaining/Sympathy-Gaining Scale
- **A** competitive
- **B** assertive
- **C** self-disciplined
- **D** self-controlled
- **E** *affectionate
- **F** *appreciated
- **G** *cared about
- **H** *tender
- **I** *kind to self (added for this study)

III Mastery-Losing/Sympathy-Losing Scale
- **A** incompetent
- **B** overly indulgent
- **C** weak
- **D** undisciplined
- **E** *forgotten
- **F** *deprived
- **G** *neglected
- **H** *not cared about
- **I** *depriving self (added for this study)

* These were reverse-coded.

Because the mastery–sympathy adjectives used in this scale are not neutral with respect to gaining–losing, the mastery–sympathy pair cannot be assessed directly. To use the scale to determine whether a participant is in the mastery or sympathy state, two steps are required. First, the participant's score on the Gaining–Losing subscale is determined. Second, the participant's score on the relevant mastery–sympathy subscale is determined. For instance, if the score is above the midpoint (the participant is considered to be gaining), then the score on the Mastery-Gaining/Sympathy-Gaining (MGSG) subscale is used. A score above the midpoint on the the Mastery-Gaining/Sympathy-Gaining subscale represents the mastery state; a score below the midpoint represents the sympathy state. If a participant's gaining–losing score is below the midpoint, the Mastery-Losing/Sympathy-Losing (MLSL) subscale is applied. A score above the midpoint on the Mastery-Losing/Sympathy-Losing subscale represents the mastery state, and a score below the midpoint represents the sympathy state. The AuMSSM, therefore, classifies each participant into one of four groups: mastery-gaining, sympathy-gaining, mastery-losing, and sympathy-losing.

Procedures

Participants were randomly assigned to respond to one of four scenarios depicting (a) success at resisting an urge to engage in an unhealthy habit, (b) failure to resist an urge to engage in an unhealthy habit, (c) success at engaging in a new health behavior, and (d) failure to engage in a new health behavior. The scenarios used in this study (see the list that follows) were similar, but not identical, to the scenarios used to develop the AuMSSM. The scenarios for this study all depicted intra-autic mastery situations in which the participant succeeded or failed at mastery. In pilot work for developing the AuMSSM, it was noted that scenarios describing situations in which individuals succeed in mastering do not always elicit memories of situations that are accompanied by positive hedonic tone. For instance, some participants might view specific mastery situations with regret (perhaps because they were allocentric at the time). In the instrument development study, the authors' interest was in eliciting memories of mastery situations in which the participants were happy about succeeding. Thus, they specified in the scenario the type of hedonic tone they were experiencing. In this study, however, part of the question had to do with what type of hedonic tone the participants had experienced during the episodes. Therefore, the scenarios in this study did not specify the hedonic tone of the participant other than to indicate success or failure during the episode. Participants were instructed to read the scenario description and to think of the last time that they, themselves, were in a similar situation. Examples of each type of situation were given. Participants were then instructed to write a brief description of the situation and to answer the questionnaire as they would have answered it during the episode they described. If participants had not actually experienced such an episode, they were asked to imagine and describe a similar experience. The instructions directed the participants to indicate whether the situation they described was actual or imagined.

Intra-Autic Mastery Scenarios Used in This Study

Urge–Success—Think about a specific instance when you succeeded in overcoming the urge to do something that you decided you shouldn't do (such as have an extra dessert, smoke a cigarette, sleep in late).

Urge–failure—Think about a specific instance when you failed to overcome the urge to do something that you decided you shouldn't do (such as have an extra dessert, smoke a cigarette, sleep in late).

New behavior–success—Think about a specific instance when you decided to start a new habit that was good for your health (such as attending an exercise session, using sunscreen, using a seat belt, eating breakfast when you usually didn't, using stress reduction techniques). Think about a specific incident when you succeeded in carrying out this habit.

New behavior–failure—Think about a specific instance when you decided to start a new habit that was good for your health (such as attending an exercise session, using sunscreen, using a seatbelt, eating breakfast when you usually didn't, using stress reduction techniques). Think about a specific incident when you failed to carry out this habit.

Data Analyses

Chi-square analyses were used to address each of the research questions. For each metamotivational pair, an initial analysis comparing the four types of scenarios with the states was carried out to determine if there were overall differences in the proportions of participants in different states across the four scenarios. Sample sizes vary because of missing data on different subscales. To address Research Question 1, which concerned differences in state as a function of success or failure, chi-square analyses compared the proportion of participants in each state who responded to success scenarios with the proportion who responded to failure scenarios. Research Questions 2 and 3 involved the interaction between the urge–new-behavior dimension and the success–fail dimension. Research Question 2 concerns the states participants were in when they succeeded at either resisting an urge or carrying out a new behavior. Research Question 3 concerns the states participants were in when they failed to either resist an urge or carry out a new behavior. Both of these questions were addressed with chi-square analyses on subsets of the cells. Separate analyses were carried out for each pair of metamotivational states.

TELIC–PARATELIC STATE

To investigate the telic–paratelic state differences as a function of scenario type, two sets of chi-square analyses were carried out. In one set, the scenarios were crossed with the serious–playful pair. In the second set of analyses, the four scenarios were crossed with the arousal-avoidance/arousal-seeking pair. Table 1 shows the number of participants classified as serious or playful for each of the four scenarios. The 2 × 4 chi-square analysis comparing the proportion of participants in serious–playful states in the four scenarios showed that there was a significant relationship between the four scenarios and the serious–playful pair, $\chi^2(3, N = 218) = 27.43$, $p < .0001$. Follow-up analyses addressing Research Question 1 revealed that success–failure was significantly related to serious–playful, $\chi^2(1, N = 218) = 11.0$, $p < .001$.

Fourteen percent of the participants responding to the success scenarios were in the paratelic state, and 33% of the participants responding to the failure scenarios were in the paratelic state. Follow-up analyses addressing Research Question 2 found no relationship between serious-minded–playful and the two types of successes. In the urge–success situation, 86% of the participants were telic; in the new-behavior–success situation, 87% of the participants were telic. Follow-up analysis addressing Research Question 3, which involved comparing the urge–failure scenario with the new-behavior–failure scenario was significant, $\chi^2(1, N = 108) = 12.59$, $p < .0004$; 16% of the participants responding to the new-behavior–failure scenario were paratelic, and 48% of the participants responding to the urge–failure scenario were paratelic. Thus, overall, failure at resisting an urge is more likely to be associated with the paratelic state than is failure to carry out a new behavior, and success at resisting an urge and at carrying out a new behavior are both associated with the telic state.

With respect to the arousal-avoidant/arousal-seeking pair, the 2 × 4 chi-square analysis relating the four scenarios to arousal-avoidant and arousal-seeking states was nonsignificant, $\chi^2(3, N = 220) = 4.73$, $p = .19$, indicating that scenarios were unrelated to the arousal-avoidant/arousal-seeking pair. Additional analyses indicated no significant differences in the arousal-avoiding/arousal-seeking pair as a function of success–fail or as a function of urge–new behavior. For all types of scenarios, over 75% of the participants were in arousal-avoidant states.

Table 1 Frequencies of Participants Classified as Serious and Playful by Scenario Type

Meta-motivational state	Urge–success	Urge–failure	New behavior–success	New behavior–failure
Serious	48	30	47	42
Playful	8	28	7	8

Table 2   Frequencies of Participants Classified as Negativistic
and Conformist by Scenario Type

Meta-motivational state	Urge–success	Urge–failure	New behavior–success	New behavior–failure
Negativistic	13	25	7	15
Conformist	44	34	46	31

NEGATIVISTIC–CONFORMIST STATE

Table 2 shows the frequencies for the negativistic–conformist states by scenario type. The 2 × 4 chi-square analysis relating the negativistic–conformist states to the four scenarios was significant, $\chi^2(3, N = 215) = 13.07$, $p < .005$. Follow-up comparisons of the success scenarios with the failure scenarios revealed a significant relationship, $\chi^2(1, N = 215) = 10.59$, $p = .001$. Only 18% of the participants responding to the success scenarios reported negativistic states, whereas 38% of the participants responding to failure scenarios reported negativistic states.

Neither the analysis comparing urge–failure with new behavior–failure nor the analysis comparing urge–success with new behavior–success was significant. Thus, success at resisting an urge and in carrying out a new behavior were uniformly associated with being in the conformist state. Resisting urges did not differ from carrying out new behaviors with respect to the negativistic–conformist pair.

MASTERY–SYMPATHY STATE

To address the research questions with respect to the mastery–sympathy state, a 4 × 4 chi-square analysis was carried out, comparing the four scenarios to the four types of mastery–sympathy states (mastery-losing, mastery-gaining, sympathy-losing, sympathy-gaining). Table 3 shows the frequencies on which this

Table 3   Frequencies of Participants Classified as Sympathy-losing, Mastery-losing, Sympathy-gaining, and Mastery-gaining by Scenario Type

Metamotivational state	Urge–success	Urge–failure	New behavior–success	New behavior–failure
Sympathy-losing	7	3	7	5
Mastery-losing	4	33	2	31
Sympathy-gaining	7	19	12	7
Mastery-gaining	36	2	35	6

analysis was based. The analysis was significant, $\chi^2(9, N = 210) = 111.18, p <$ .0001. When the success scenarios were compared with the failure scenarios across the four types of mastery–sympathy states, the analysis was also significant, $\chi^2(3, N = 210) = 99.38, p < .001$. As expected, the majority (68%) of the participants responding to success scenarios were categorized as mastery-gaining, and the majority (60%) of the participants responding to the failure scenarios were categorized as mastery-losing. As expected, when mastery-losing and mastery-gaining states were collapsed to a mastery category and when the sympathy-gaining and sympathy-losing states were collapsed to a sympathy category, there was no significant relationship between mastery and sympathy and success–fail. This finding indicates that it is important to know whether the participant is losing or gaining during the episode. The participants in the failure scenarios were expected to be categorized as losing and the participants responding to the success scenarios, as gaining. Surprisingly, a total of 34 (32%) of the participants responding to failure scenarios were categorized as gaining, and a total of 14 (13%) participants responding to the success scenarios were categorized as losing.

To address Research Question 2, comparing the types of success scenarios for the mastery–sympathy pair, two 2 × 2 analyses were carried out. The first of these analyses included the 90 participants responding to the success scenarios who were categorized by the AuMSSM as gaining; the second analysis included the 14 participants responding to success scenarios who were categorized as losing. For the 90 participants classified as gaining, the analysis comparing urge success with new-behavior–success scenarios was nonsignificant. The urge-success and new-behavior–success scenarios did not differ with respect to whether the participants were in mastery-gaining or sympathy-gaining states. At least 74.5% of the participants in either type of situation were categorized as mastery-gaining. In the second analysis, a 2 × 2 Fisher's exact test was carried out with the 14 participants responding to success scenarios who were categorized as losing. Urge–success scenarios did not differ significantly from new-behavior–success scenarios on the mastery-losing/sympathy-losing pair. However, it should be noted that of the 8 participants in this analysis who were classified as sympathy-losing, 7 were participants who were responding to urge-success situations. Therefore, for some participants, succeeding at resisting an urge is more likely to be accompanied by the negative feelings of being deprived and neglected than by positive feelings of self-discipline and self-control.

Although the success scenarios did not differ with respect to the mastery–sympathy pair, exploratory analyses revealed that they did differ with respect to hedonic tone. A 2 × 2 chi-square analysis comparing participants classified as gaining with participants classified as losing on the two types of success scenario was significant, $\chi^2(1, N = 104) = 4.6, p = .03$. Twenty percent of the participants successfully resisting urges were classified as losing, whereas only 6% of the participants successfully carrying out new behaviors were classified as losing. Therefore, succeeding at carrying out new behaviors was more likely to be associated with positive hedonic tone than was success at resisting urges.

To address Research Question 3, comparing the failure scenarios, two 2×2 chi-square analyses were carried out. In the first analysis, which included the 72 participants responding to the failure scenarios who were classified by the AuMSSM as losing, urge–failure scenarios did not differ from new-behavior–failure scenarios on the mastery-losing/sympathy-losing pair. At least 86% of these participants were classified as mastery-losing. The second analysis of the 34 participants responding to failure scenarios who were classified as gaining showed significant differences between the urge–failure scenarios and the new-behavior–failure scenarios on the mastery-gaining/sympathy-gaining pair, $\chi^2(1, N = 34) = 6.0$, $p < .01$. Ninety percent of the participants in the urge–failure category were in the sympathy-gaining state, and only 54% of those in the new-behavior–failure scenario were in the sympathy-gaining state. Thus, participants who failed to resist an urge were more likely to report feeling tender and kind to self than were participants who failed at carrying out a new behavior.

DISCUSSION OF STUDY FINDINGS

This study explored the metamotivational consequences of attempting to change health-related behaviors. The health-related behaviors participants reported in this study varied according to whether the behavior involved resisting an urge to carry out an old behavior or succeeding in carrying out a new behavior. Urges that participants resisted or succumbed to included urges to smoke, eat, and have sex, though the urge to eat was the most frequently reported urge. New behaviors included exercise, seatbelt use, and sunscreen use, though exercise was the most frequently reported new behavior.

In answer to the first research question concerning which metamotivational variables are associated with success at changing behavior, the study showed that success was related to the serious-minded and conformist states and failure was associated with the paratelic and negativistic states. These results are similar to the findings in the first author's previous work on smoking cessation, which showed that lapsing during a highly tempting situation was preceded by paratelic or negativistic states, or by both (O'Connell et al., 1990; Potocky et al., 1991). As expected, the relationship of success to the mastery–sympathy pair was more complicated and depended on whether the participants were on the losing or gaining end of the gain–loss continuum.

With respect to Research Question 2, involving the comparison of situations where participants were successful at resisting urges with situations in which participants were successful at carrying out new behaviors, the results of this study suggest that the metamotivational consequences of succeeding are similar for both types of behavior. Within success situations, resisting urges was not different from carrying out a new behavior with respect to the telic–paratelic pair, the negativistic–conformist pair, the mastery-gaining/sympathy-gaining pair, or the mastery/sympathy-losing pair (though the latter had only 14 participants in the analysis). Participants who succeeded in resisting urges and carrying out new behaviors were in telic, conformist, and mastery-gaining states. However, there was a suggestion in the data that succeeding at resisting an urge was more likely to be accompanied by negative hedonic tone than was succeeding at carrying out a new behavior. Thus, success at resisting an urge is not always accompanied by pleasant feelings.

With respect to Research Question 3, involving the comparison of situations where participants failed at resisting urges with situations in which participants failed at carrying out new behaviors, findings provide evidence that the experience of giving up old habits differs from the experience of adopting new habits. Failure to resist an urge was more likely to result in paratelic states than was failure to carry out a new behavior; in addition, failure to resist an urge was more likely to result in sympathy-gaining states than was failure to carry out new behaviors. Within the failure situations, resisting urges was no different from carrying out new behaviors with respect to the negativistic–conformist pair or the mastery-losing/sympathy-losing pair. Thus, overcoming urges is associated with different metamotivational outcomes than is carrying out new behaviors. Almost half of the participants who failed at resisting urges were in playful states, whereas only 16% of those failing to carry out new behaviors were in paratelic states. Thus, being in playful states is associated with succumbing to urges. In addition, rather than experiencing a failure to resist an urge as a humiliating sign of weakness, a sizable number of those who fail experience it as pleasant feelings of being cared for and kind to self. This outcome is understandable. Failure to resist an urge results in the opportunity to engage in a valued and gratifying behavior, whereas failure to carry out a new behavior usually leads to few immediate consequences.

Although this study was conceptualized as a report of the metamotivational consequences of succeeding and failing at acquiring health habits, to the extent that the participants maintained the same metamotivational state before and after the success and failure experiences, the states reported by the participants may also reflect antecedents to success and failure. The fact that the states resulting from urge–failure scenarios are similar to the states preceding smoking lapses provides evidence for the argument that participants may remain in the same metamotivational states before, during, and immediately after the success–failure episode. Thus, in addition to showing the metamotivational consequences of success and failure, this study may give clues to the metamotivational states in which participants are particularly vulnerable to failure.

CONCLUSION

Taking into account its limitations, this study does provide initial evidence that specific instances of two types of health behaviors yield different experiential outcomes. These outcomes give clues to the problems with long-term behavior change. Even if one does experience success in a specific instance, the success may not be accompanied by pleasant hedonic tone. Furthermore, failure is sometimes accompanied by pleasant hedonic tone, especially if the behavior involves resisting urges. The challenge for health promotion advocates is to help clients to reframe their successes and their failures. A previous study of smoking cessation (O'Connell et al., 1995) showed that sympathy states usually lead to lapsing in highly tempting situations. However, sympathy states are not necessarily associated with failure to resist an urge. It is possible to see resisting an urge as a way of nurturing oneself, that is, to be associated with a sympathy-gaining outcome. It is likewise possible to see engaging in exercise as a way to be kind to oneself (lower stress, feel better, etc). In fact, in this study, 21% of the participants responding to success scenarios were categorized as sympathy-gaining. Thus, for some participants, succeeding in engaging in health behaviors is seen more as a way to nurture themselves than as an exercise in self-control. This study illustrates the usefulness of reversal theory constructs for understanding changes in health behavior. Regarding health behavior as a way to nurture oneself will maximize the possibility of engaging in those behaviors during sympathy states. Regarding health behavior as a way to achieve self-control and other pleasant mastery outcomes will maximize the possibility of engaging in those behaviors during mastery states. The ability to regard health behaviors as having positive outcomes in both mastery states and sympathy states will maximize the possibility of long-term behavior change.

REFERENCES

Apter, M. J., & Smith, K. C. P. (1985). Experiencing personal relationships. In M. J. Apter, D. Fontana, & S. Murgatroyd (Eds.), *Reversal theory: Applications and developments* (pp. 161–178). Cardiff, Wales: University College Cardiff Press.

Brownell, K. D., Marlatt, G. A., Lichtenstein, E., & Wilson, G. T. (1986). Understanding and preventing relapse. *American Psychologist, 41,* 765–782.

Calhoun, J. E., & O'Connell, K. A. (1995, July). Construct validity of the Telic/Paratelic State Instrument: A measure of reversal theory constructs. Presented at the Seventh International Conference on Reversal Theory, Melbourne, Victoria, Australia.

Cook, M. R., Gerkovich, M. M., O'Connell, K. A., & Potocky, M. (1995). Reversal theory constructs and cigarette availability predict lapse early in smoking cessation. *Research in Nursing & Health, 18,* 217–224.

Cook, M. R., Gerkovich, M. M., Potocky, M., & O'Connell, K. A. (1993). Instruments for the assessment of reversal theory states. *Patient Education and Counseling, 22,* 99–106.

O'Connell, K. A. (1993). A lexicon for the mastery/sympathy and autic/alloic states. In J. H. Kerr, S. J. Murgatroyd, & M. J. Apter (Eds.), *Advances in reversal theory* (pp. 53–65). Amsterdam: Swets & Zeitlinger.

O'Connell, K. A., & Apter, M. J. (1993). Mastery and sympathy: Conceptual elaboration of the transactional states. In J. H. Kerr, S. J. Murgatroyd, & M. J. Apter (Eds.), *Advances in reversal theory* (pp. 41–51). Amsterdam: Swets & Zeitlinger.

O'Connell, K. A., Cook, M. R., Gerkovich, M. M., Potocky, M., & Swan, G. E. (1990). Reversal theory and smoking: A state-based approach to ex-smokers' highly tempting situations. *Journal of Consulting and Clinical Psychology, 58,* 489–494.

O'Connell, K., Gerkovich, M. M., & Cook, M. R. (1995). Reversal theory's mastery and sympathy states in smoking cessation. *Image: Journal of Nursing Scholarship, 27,* 311–316.

Potocky, M., Gerkovich, M. M., O'Connell, K. A., & Cook, M. R. (1991). State-outcome consistency in smoking relapse crises: A reversal theory approach. *Journal of Consulting and Clinical Psychology, 59,* 351—353.

Popkess-Vawter, S., & Wendel, S. (1995, July). *Motivations for overeating in overweight and normal weight females.* Presented at the Seventh International Conference on Reversal Theory, Melbourne, Victoria, Australia.

14

Humor as a Form of Coping

Sven Svebak and Rod A. Martin

Humor can be seen as a paratelic form of coping with everyday hassles, frustrations, and stressful events. The defining characteristics of humorous cognitive synergies are presented, and a person–situation interaction model is given to illustrate contingencies that may facilitate and inhibit the experience of mirthful laughter. Results from an empirical test of reversal theory hypotheses in relation to mirthful laughter are presented, and studies of central nervous processing modes related to humor appreciation are also reviewed. An overview is given of methods for the assessment of individual differences in sense of humor that were used in empirical studies reviewed in this chapter. The main findings from these studies are presented to evaluate the potential for sense of humor as a mediator of health and moderator of adverse effects of stressors on mood, bodily complaints, and immune function. Overall, these findings are supportive of the conclusion that (a) sense of humor exerts a buffering effect on the relation between stressors and negative moods and that this effect may also involve the mediation of positive moods and (b) there is little support for any direct effect of sense of humor on mood and psychobiological health outcome variables, but a buffering effect of sense of humor is clearly supported in conjunction with daily hassles, frustrations, and stressful life events. Thus, sense of humor interacts with stressors to moderate their effects on moods, complaints, and immune function.

Mirthful laughter is accompanied by a wide range of psychobiological changes. These include respiratory changes, facial muscle contractions, postural changes that sometimes may develop into generalized muscle cramps, circulatory changes resulting in the reddening of the face, and sympathetic activation that provokes sweat. All these changes are indications of catabolic changes of the metabolic activity in the body. The inherent pleasure in mirthful laughter is an excellent example of the shortcomings of optimal arousal theory. This theory suggests that medium levels of arousal give rise to pleasant experiences, whereas low as well as high levels of arousal give rise to the experience of some kind of dis-pleasure (e.g., boredom and anxiety, respectively; see, e.g., Berlyne, 1972). Data against this inverted-U formulation with humor appreciation existed already in the 1970s (Godkewitsch, 1972; Langevin & Day, 1972). In contrast, reversal theory posits that high levels of arousal are experienced as enjoyable (excite-ment) when one is in the paratelic state and give rise to unpleasant emotion (anxiety) only when one is in the telic state (see Chapter 1).

One example of the difference between these two theories, along a slightly different line of thinking, is reflected in the cultivation of low arousal, such as in the clinical use of biofeedback and relaxation training (Stoyva & Budzynski, 1974). This approach may be appropriate for the lowering of high arousal in the anxious patient. However, it is adaptive only on the premise that the patient is in the telic state or is telic state–dominant and experiencing enduring high levels of arousal, which means anxiety or anger in that state (depending on the coinci-dence of the conformist or negativistic states, respectively). Conversely, Svebak and Stoyva (1980) suggested that some forms of high arousal might even be beneficial to health. Perhaps the most popular current example is the prevailing view that physical exercise promotes health. However, the emotional conse-quences of physical exercise are not always those of pleasant emotions (Kerr & Svebak, 1994). In contrast, individuals with high sense of humor may have a disposition toward cognitive appraisal of hassles, frustrations, and other stres-sors in everyday life that help them cope with potentially unpleasant arousal in ways that transform into mirthfulness. If so, this way of coping may be benefi-cial to one's emotional life, general well-being, and physical health.

THE NATURE OF COGNITIVE APPRAISAL IN HUMOR

One of the chapters in the original book on reversal theory by Apter (1982) dealt exclusively with the cognitive processing that is peculiar to humor. Ac-cording to Apter, humor is an example of what he called *cognitive synergy*. He defined this as the bringing together in consciousness of opposite qualities in relation to a given identity (person, object, or situation). In the case of humor, these opposites exist at two levels. One of these is the level of reality, and the other is the level of appearance. That is, what at first appears to be reality is revealed to be only appearance, and an opposite quality is disclosed to be the "real" reality. Furthermore, the reality that is disclosed in this way is always in some sense "less," for example, less powerful, less socially approved, less pres-tigious, or less valuable than the one that the identity purported to be.

Apter (1982) provided many examples of such humor synergies (as well as synergies of other kinds, e.g., aesthetic synergies). Some of these humor examples related to comic personalities where incompatible qualities are endur-ing and others to jokes that depend on more ephemeral characteristics. It is beyond the purpose of this chapter to present this analysis in detail. Suffice it to say that the ability of an individual to interpret real-life experiences in a humorous way involves the potential for appraisal and reappraisal in such a manner that seemingly threatening events and circumstances come to be construed as less genuinely threatening than they initially appeared to be. Some recent evidence that is largely supportive of this reversal theory analysis of humor can be found in Wyer and Collins (1992).

The mechanism of humor, according to Apter (1982), involves two components: The first increases the level of felt arousal temporarily, and the second brings about a switch to the paratelic state. Or if the individual is already in the paratelic state, humor works to maintain that state. The very rapid telic-to-paratelic switch means that the increase of arousal due to humor is pleasant rather than unpleasant. As in other types of synergy, the inherent puzzle itself induces arousal, and the subsequent attempt to make sense of puzzles also increases arousal. On top of these arousal-inducing consequences of humor comes the expressive behavior of laughter, which further increases arousal as a result of the motor changes. One characteristic of the paratelic state is that high levels of arousal are preferred and experienced as some kind of pleasant excitement (see Chapter 1).

THE PSYCHOBIOLOGY OF HUMOR APPRECIATION

So far, it has been pointed out that humor appreciation is a particular type of cognitive process, involving real or apparent synergies, and that the paratelic state provides the metamotivational state where the arousal-inducing consequences of this process will be enjoyed. Situational contingencies are also important in the way they may provide cues that facilitate or inhibit the expression of mirthfulness or even the appropriateness of the paratelic state. Svebak and Apter (1987) reported evidence indicating that even telic-dominant individuals reverse to the paratelic state when watching a comedy and that paratelic-dominant individuals remain in their dominant state. Moreover, measures of respiration provided evidence for laughter (see Svebak, 1975, for operational criteria). Ratings were derived for felt as well as preferred levels of arousal and for telic–paratelic state in the laboratory entertainment situation.

The results from Svebak and Apter (1987) confirmed the hypothesis that humorous material tends to induce the paratelic state even in extremely telic state–dominant individuals and that frequency of laughter in the paratelic state is positively correlated with degree of felt arousal ($r = .70$, $p < .01$) and with preferred level of arousal ($r = .44$, $p < .05$). In contrast to predictions by optimal arousal theory, these findings indicated a linear rather than a ditonic relation of hedonic tone to felt arousal in the paratelic state. By and large, the data encourage the exploration of humor as a particular form of coping with life stress.

There are a few studies of the relationship between brain damage and humor appreciation. Bihrle, Brownell, Powelson, and Gardner (1986) studied the ability to perceive humorous messages among 17 patients with left hemisphere damage, 10 patients with right hemisphere damage, and 10 healthy control participants. In both groups with brain damage, some had damage in the frontal and others in the parietal and occipital or temporal areas. All participants were exposed to a test of ability to organize sequences of four pictures to make the best possible humorous "story" in each case. Results indicated that right hemisphere damage caused poor coherence although a sense of surprise was maintained, whereas a left hemisphere damage was detrimental to the sense of surprise although the sense of coherence was maintained. In both cases, a reduction of the sense of humor was apparent, but for different reasons.

The results reported by Bihrle et al. (1986) may support the assumption that sense of humor is one of the most advanced cognitive-processing modes in the human brain and that talents located in both hemispheres are called on in order to successfully perform the humor synergy process. Svebak (1982) reported electroencephalographic (EEG) evidence indicating that a sequence of mirthful laughter when watching a comedy elicits a subsequent increase in the coordination of the alpha patterns in the right and left hemisphere occipital lobes. This finding is interesting in light of several reports on the increase of right hemisphere EEG variability, as compared with that of the left hemisphere, and that this kind of dissociation of the right hemisphere is a characteristic of depression (d'Elia & Perris, 1973; Goldstein, Temple, & Pollack, 1976). In a Darwinian sense, when these brain findings are taken together, the humor-processing capacity of the brain appears to involve a coordination of the brain hemispheres. This is the opposite of what is seen in depression. The healthy human brain has been formed to incorporate a potential for concerted action in humor cognitions to facilitate survival of the human species.

Lefcourt and Martin (1986) reported a series of studies in support of the idea that sense of humor is an antidote to adversity, although reversal theory was not the major theoretical perspective in their book. The evidence in support of humor as being appreciated specifically in the paratelic state provided a good reason for looking also at results from studies that were not initiated to explicitly test reversal theory assumptions. Therefore, those studies in which Lefcourt and Martin reported mood disturbance related to life stress and sense of humor are reviewed after presenting methods for assessing individual differences of sense of humor.

MEASURES OF SENSE OF HUMOR

One of the earliest survey methods for measuring individual differences in sense of humor was published in 1974 as the Sense of Humor Questionnaire (SHQ; Svebak, 1974). This 21-item measure was designed to assess three different aspects of sense of humor with 7 items on each. The first subscale was termed Meta-Message Sensitivity and asks about one's habitual readiness to perceive humorous messages, that is, the sensitivity toward cognitive humor synergies. An example from this subscale would be "I can usually find something comical, witty, or humorous in most situations." The second subscale was termed Personal Liking of Humor, and items ask about the degree to which participants value humor in their lives, including humorous others and participating in situations that provide opportunities for humor and laughter. An item in this subscale is "It is my impression that those who try to be funny really do it to hide their lack of self-confidence" (disagreement scores high). The third subscale has 7 items on readiness for emotional expression (Emotional Expressiveness). One item in this section is "I appreciate people who tolerate all kinds of emotional expression." Martin and his associates (e.g., Lefcourt & Martin, 1986) found low internal consistency for items on this latter subscale (a = .25), whereas the two former subscales yielded acceptable alpha scores on internal consistency of items. The Emotional Expressiveness subscale has not been used in health-related studies involving this scale, although a revised version of the SHQ scale is underway and may prove more encouraging. In contrast, the two former subscales, and the Social Liking subscale in particular, have been used in several recent studies.

The Situational Humor Response Questionnaire (SHRQ) was constructed by Martin and Lefcourt (1984) to assess individual differences in sense of humor in terms of the frequency with which they respond with mirth in a variety of situations. One of the 21 items is "If you were shopping by yourself in a distant city and you unexpectedly saw an acquaintance from school (or work), how have you responded or how would you respond?" (5-point scale for scoring, ranging from *I would probably not have bothered to speak to the person*, scoring 1, to *I would have laughed heartily with the person*, scoring 5).

The Coping Humor Scale (CHS) is a seven-item scale that has also proved to yield interesting data in relation to stress outcomes (Martin & Lefcourt, 1973). One item example is "I often lose my sense of humor when I'm having problems." (The scale is scored on 4-point Likert scales and with alpha scores in the .60 to 70 range; see Lefcourt & Martin, 1986).

SENSE OF HUMOR AND CONSEQUENCES OF STRESS

Stress Tolerance

A three-step procedure was implemented in the series of studies on buffering effects of sense of humor on the relation between stress and mood as well as health outcome (see Figure 1). Step 1 examines the simple correlation between stress and negative outcomes. The obvious fact that stress must be involved in a study of the potential for sense of humor to buffer consequences of stress does not preclude the possibility that a Step 2 effect may also be observed: Sense of humor may have a direct effect on mood and health outcomes independent of the potential for stressors to have detrimental consequences. In Step 3, the moderating effect of sense of humor is tested by use of the product of (lack of) sense of humor and stress exposure. This buffering effect, when significant, means that sense of humor is an antidote to adversity only when life is stressful.

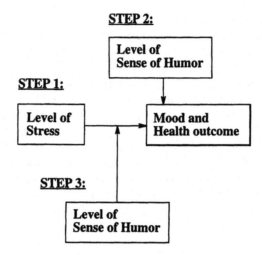

Figure 1 An illustration of the procedure for testing the role of sense of humor as a potential buffer against detrimental effects of stressors on mood, bodily complaints, and biological mechanisms involved in disease processes. Note that Steps 1 and 2 are independent direct effects on outcome variables, whereas Step 3 represents the moderating effect due to interaction of stressors and (lack of) sense of humor in relation to outcome variables.

The nature of the hypotheses underlying each of these three steps is illustrated in Figure 2. Statistical analyses, according to this three-step format, are performed by use of a hierarchical multiple regression procedure.

The pioneering three-step study was reported by Martin and Lefcourt (1983), who assessed life stress by use of the Negative Life Events scale (NLE; Sandler & Lakey, 1982), and sense of humor was assessed by use of the SHRQ, SHQ, and CHS. Mood disturbance was measured by the Profile of Mood States (POMS;

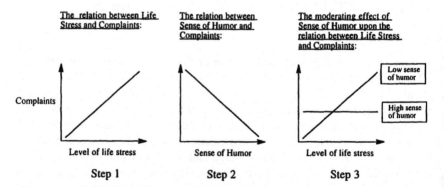

Figure 2 Illustrations of the hypotheses underlying each of the three steps (see Figure 1) in hierarchical multiple regression analyses of relations between stressful life events, sense of humor, and negative outcomes (e.g., bodily complaints).

McNair, Lorr, & Droppleman, 1971). Fifty-six university students took part, and results confirmed that significant buffering effects (Step 3 effects) were found for sense of humor on the relation between negative life events and mood disturbance. This effect was significant when sense of humor was measured by the SHRQ ($p < .05$) and SHQ (Liking of Humor subscale, $p < .05$), as well as the CHS ($p < .05$). Mood disturbance was less marked with stress among individuals who scored high on these measures of sense of humor (see Martin & Lefcourt, 1983, for details).

In another study, Martin and his colleagues examined the role of sense of humor in moderating the relationship between negative life events and positive rather than negative moods (Kuiper, Martin, & Dance, 1992). In this study, participants completed a mood measure each day for 2 weeks. Hierarchical multiple regression analyses were used to predict mean positive mood scores from negative life events and the humor scales. As in the previous studies with negative moods, the results revealed significant interactions of negative life events with the CHS, the SHRQ, and the SHQ (Meta-Message Sensitivity subscale) in predicting positive moods. Further examination of these interactions revealed that participants with low humor scores had a strong negative correlation between the number of negative life events and the level of self-reported positive moods. In contrast, those with high humor scores actually showed a slightly positive correlation between these variables, suggesting that high humor participants may actually be somewhat invigorated by experiencing stressful events, rather than having a reduction in positive moods. This pattern of results is again consistent with the predictions of reversal theory, with increased stress (and, presumably, arousal) being associated with more positive moods in individuals with a greater proclivity to humor (a paratelic activity).

Using a somewhat different approach to investigate the stress-moderating effects of humor, Hudak, Dale, and Hudak (1991) made use of the SHRQ in a study examining the effects of watching a humorous videotape versus a nonhumorous videotape on participants' threshold for discomfort when exposed to transcutaneous end nerve stimulation. A main effect was found for the experimental manipulation, with participants watching the humorous videotape showing an increase in threshold for discomfort and those watching a nonhumorous videotape having a decreased threshold. Interestingly, these results appeared to be largely due to participants with low SHRQ scores showing a particularly strong drop in their discomfort threshold in the nonhumorous condition. Thus, when provided with a humorous videotape to watch, participants with either high or low humor scores showed similar increases in discomfort threshold. However, when no humor was provided, those participants who did not normally laugh and smile as much (as reflected in low scores on the SHRQ) showed a strong decrease in threshold, whereas those who do normally laugh and smile in a wide variety of situations showed a much smaller decline in threshold.

A similar type of design was used by Yovetich, Dale, and Hudak (1990) in examining the effects of humor on the incubation of threat effect. Participants listened to either a humorous or a nonhumorous audiotape or no tape while waiting 12 min for an expected painful electric shock. Heart rate and electromyograms were monitored, and self-reports of anxiety were obtained. The results revealed that participants listening to the humorous tape showed significantly fewer indices of anxiety as the expected shock approached than did those in the other two conditions. In addition, scores on the SHRQ interacted with these effects. Overall, participants with lower SHRQ scores showed a greater increase in anxiety as the shock approached. Moreover, participants with low SHRQ scores appeared to benefit particularly from the humorous tape, whereas those with high SHRQ scores had similar anxiety and physiological levels in all three conditions. Thus, as in the study described previously, participants who do not normally laugh and smile as often (i.e., low SHRQ scorers) are more adversely affected when no humor is provided and benefit more from the provision of humorous stimuli, whereas those who do normally show mirthful behaviors in their daily lives (i.e., high SHRQ scorers) appear to maintain a more even disposition regardless of whether humorous material is provided for them.

Health outcomes

The three-step procedure, as described above, adopted in the studies by Martin and his associates, as described above, was replicated by Svebak and his students in Norway, using a somewhat different measure of life stress (the Tension and Effort Stress Inventory, as described in Chapter 5; see Svebak, 1993, where the main findings from this study are reviewed).

The replication study (see Svebak, 1993) included the SHQ Liking of Humor subscale as well as a survey on common complaints related to the skeletal muscles, gastrointestinal tract, and cardiovascular, respiratory, and immune systems (the Ursin Health Inventory; Ursin, Endresen, & Ursin, 1988). Seventy-five university students in different subject fields were recruited for this study, and all survey measures were completed approximately 4 weeks before an important exam. The results, which are given in Table 1, confirmed a direct effect of stress on complaints attributed to the skeletal muscles, upper gastrointestinal tract as well as lower, cardiorespiratory systems, and immune-related functions. Interestingly, buffering effects of sense of humor were found in relation to all groups of complaints except for the overall score on cardiorespiratory complaints (dyspnea, pounding heart, etc.; see Table 1). Thus, the results supported the hypothesis that individuals with a stronger sense of humor are less likely to experience such problems when confronted by stressful life demands. Furthermore, most of the research to date has shown an interaction between stress and humor in predicting physical symptoms, Carroll and Shmidt (1992) found a significant negative correlation between scores on the SHRQ and a 13-item illness symptom inventory ($r = -.34$). This means that increased humor and laughter were associated with decreased symptoms of illness, independent of levels of stress.

Martin and Dobbin (1988) measured salivary immunoglobulin A (IgA) and,

Table 1   Hierarchical Multiple Regression Analyses for the Association Between Different Types of Complaints and Stress Due to Work, Family, and Finance; Sense of Humor; and the Product of Stress and (Relative Lack of) Sense of Humor

Complaint	Total r^2	df	F score	F change	p value
Muscles					
Stress (Step 1)	.31	1, 53	5.44		.024
Humor (Step 2)	.43	1, 52		5.58	.022
Humor × Stress (Step 3)	.50	1, 51		4.95	.031
Upper gastrointestinal					
Stress (Step 1)	.48	1, 56	16.94		.0001
Humor (Step 2)	.52	1, 55		2.54	ns
Humor × Stress (Step 3)	.77	1, 54		43.13	.0001
Lower gastrointestinal					
Stress (Step 1)	.33	1, 55	6.89		.011
Humor (Step 2)	.37	1, 54		3.21	ns
Humor × Stress (Step 3)	.60	1, 53		19.23	.0001
Cardiorespiratory					
Stress (Step 1)	.30	1, 56	5.71		.02
Humor (Step 2)	.38	1, 55		3.21	(.07)
Humor × Stress (Step 3)	.38	1, 54		0.02	ns
Immune-related					
Stress (Step 1)	.31	1, 55	6.00		.018
Humor (Step 2)	.35	1, 54		1.34	ns
Humor × Stress (Step 3)	.54	1, 53		13.17	.0006

Adapted from Svebak, 1993.

thus, extended this three-step procedure for the study of moderating effects of sense of humor into the field of immune functions. Thirty participants were recruited for their study, and IgA was estimated from 5-ml saliva samples. After samples were obtained, participants completed the sense of humor questionnaires (SHRQ, CHS, SHQ) as well as the Daily Hassles Scale (Kanner, Coyne, Schaffer, & Lazarus, 1981). It was noted in Chapter 6 that this immunoglobulin is an antibody primarily located within the secretory fluids of the human body. It is an important defense against antigens in the upper respiratory tract as well as in the gastrointestinal tract.

The major findings from this study are summarized in Table 2, where it can be seen that the moderating effect of the interaction between hassles and (low) sense of humor on secretory IgA was significant and, therefore, explained a unique proportion of the variance in IgA scores beyond that which could be attributed to hassles alone. None of the sense-of-humor measures provided any significant direct (Step 2) effect on secretory IgA. In general, for individuals with low sense of humor, high levels of daily hassles were associated with low levels of IgA. In contrast, for individuals with high levels of sense of humor,

Table 2   Hierarchical Multiple Regression Analyses for the Association Between Salivary Immunoglobulin A and Hassles, Sense of Humor as Measured by Three Different Scales, and the Product of Stress and (Relative Lack of) Sense of Humor

Variable	Total r^2	df	F change	p value
Hassles (Step 1)	.13	1, 31	4.53	.05
SHRQ (Step 2)	.18	1, 30	1.92	ns
H × SHRQ (Step 3)	.28	1, 29	4.17	.05
Hassles (Step 1)	.10	1, 34	3.88	.06
CBS (Step 2)	.12	1, 33	0.65	ns
H × CBS (Step 3)	.24	1, 32	4.87	.05
Hassles (Step 1)	.10	1, 33	3.68	.06
SHQ-M (Step 2)	.14	1, 32	1.35	ns
H × SHQ-M (Step 3)	.31	1, 31	7.88	.01

Note. SHRQ = Situational Humor Response Questionnaire; CHS = Coping Humor Scale; SHQ-M = Sense of Humor Questionnaire (Metamessage Sensitivity Subscale). Adapted from "Sense of Humor, Hassles and Immunoglobulin A: Evidence for a Stress-Moderating Effect of Humor," by R. A. Martin and J. P. Dobbin, 1988, *International Journal of Psychiatry in Medicine, 18.*

there was no systematic effect of daily hassles on concentration of secretory IgA (see Table 2).

Dillon, Minchoff, and Baker (1985) administered the CHS and also obtained saliva samples from a small group of participants ($N = 9$). The saliva samples were subsequently assayed for levels of secretory immunoglobulin A. The results showed a strong correlation ($r = .75$) between CHS scores and IgA levels, indicating that participants with greater self-reported tendency to make use of humor in coping with stress had higher levels of this component of immunity.

In a subsequent study, Dillon and Totten (1989) studied a group of 17 women just before they gave birth and 2 months postdelivery. These participants completed the CHS and also provided saliva and breast milk samples that were assayed for IgA. As in the previous study, CHS scores were found to be highly related to salivary IgA levels ($r = .61$), but not to the IgA levels in breast milk. In addition, mothers who reported a greater likelihood of using humor to cope with life stress, as measured by the CHS, experienced significantly fewer upper respiratory infections ($r = -.51$) during the 2 months after delivery, as did their babies ($r = -.58$).

CONCLUSION

When all these findings are taken together, they provide support for several conclusions. One is that the reversal theory alternative to the idea of an inverted-U relationship (i.e., optimal arousal) is a better conceptualization of data on the relationship between arousal and hedonic tone and that mirthful laughter is a form of enjoyment of high arousal in the paratelic state. These findings also suggest that the vital survival value of the sense of humor is dependent on a central nervous system capacity for coordinated right–left hemisphere processing mode. It also provides evidence for the importance of applying a sensitive procedure in the study of the potential for sense of humor to buffer the negative consequences of stressors on mood and health. The three-step hierarchical multiple regression approach has yielded several sets of results in independent studies where the buffering capacity of sense of humor has been confirmed, in relation to mood disturbance, bodily complaints, and immune function (IgA).

REFERENCES

Apter, M. J. (1982). *The experience of motivation: The theory of psychological reversals.* London: Academic Press.

Berlyne, D. E. (1972). Humor and its kin. In J. H. Goldstein & P. E. McGhee (Eds.), *The psychology of humor* (pp. 43–60). New York: Academic Press.

Bihrle, A. M., Brownell, H. H., Powelson, J. A., & Gardner, H. (1986). Comprehension of humorous and nonhumorous materials by left and right brain-damaged patients. *Brain and Cognition, 5,* 399–411.

Carroll, J. L., & Shmidt, J. L. (1992). Correlation between humorous coping style and health. *Psychological Reports, 70,* 402.

d'Elia, G., & Perris, C. (1973). Cerebral function dominance and depression. *Acta Psychiatrica Scandinavica, 49,* 191–197.

Dillon, K. M., Minchoff, B., & Baker, K. H. (1985). Positive emotional states and enhancement of the immune system. *International Journal of Psychiatry in Medicine, 15,* 13–18.

Dillon, K. M., & Totten, M. C. (1989). Psychological factors, immunocompetence, and health of breast-feeding mothers and their infants. *Journal of Genetic Psychology, 150,* 155–162.

Godkewitsch, M. (1972). The relationship between arousal potential and funniness of jokes. In J. H. Goldstein & P. E. McGhee (Eds.), *The psychology of humor* (pp. 143–158). New York: Academic Press.

Goldstein, L., Temple, R. J., & Pollack, I. W. (1976). EEG and clinical assessment of subjects with drug abuse problems. *Research Communication in Psychology, Psychiatry and Behavior, 1,* 193–210.

Hudak, D. A., Dale, J. A., & Hudak, M. A. (1991). Effects of humorous stimuli and sense of humor on discomfort. *Psychological Reports, 69,* 779–786.

Kanner, A. D., Coyne, J. C., Schaffer, C., & Lazarus, R. S. (1981). Comparison of two modes of stress measurement: Daily Hassles and Uplifts versus Major Life Events. *Journal of Behavioral Medicine, 4,* 1–39.

Kerr, J., & Svebak, S. (1994). The acute effects of participation in sport on mood: The importance of level of "antagonistic physical interaction." *Personality and Individual Differences, 16,* 159–166.

Kuiper, N. A., Martin, R. A., & Dance, K. A. (1992). Sense of humour and enhanced quality of life. *Personality and Individual Differences 13,* 1273–1283.

Langevin, R., & Day, H. I. (1972). Physiological correlates. In J. H. Goldstein & P. E. McGhee (Eds.), *The psychology of humor* (pp. 129–142). New York: Academic Press.

Lefcourt, H. M., & Martin, R. A. (1986). *Humor and life stress: antidote to adversity.* New York: Springer Verlag.

Martin, R. A., & Dobbin, J. P. (1988). Sense of humor, hassles and immunoglobulin A: Evidence for a stress-moderating effect of humor. *International Journal of Psychiatry in Medicine, 18*, 93–105.

Martin, R. A., & Lefcourt, H. M. (1983). The sense of humor as a moderator of the relationship between stressors and moods. *Journal of Personality and Social Psychology, 45*, 1313–1324.

Martin, R. A., & Lefcourt, H. M. (1984). Situational Humor Response Questionnaire: Quantitative measure of sense of humor. *Journal of Personality and Social Psychology, 47*, 145–155.

McNair, D. M., Lorr, M., & Droppleman, L. F. (1971). *The Profile of Mood States.* San Diego: Educational and Industrial Testing Service.

Sandler, I. N., & Lakey, B. (1982). Locus of control as a stress moderator: The role of control perceptions and social support. *American Journal of Consulting and Clinical Psychology, 10*, 65–80.

Stoyva, J., & Budzynski, T. H. (1974). Cultivated low arousal—An anti-stress response? In L. V. DiCara (Ed.), *Recent advances in limbic and autonomic nervous system research* (pp. 369–394). New York: Plenum Press.

Svebak, S. (1974). Revised questionnaire on the sense of humor. *Scandinavian Journal of Psychology, 15*, 328–331.

Svebak, S. (1975). Respiratory patterns as predictors of laughter. *Psychophysiology, 12*, 62–65.

Svebak, S. (1982). The effect of mirthfulness upon amount of discordant right-left occipital EEG alpha. *Motivation and Emotion, 6*, 133–147.

Svebak, S. (1993). The development of the Tension and Effort Stress Inventory (TESI). In J. H. Kerr, S. Murgatroyd, & M. J. Apter (Eds.), *Advances in reversal theory* (pp. 189–204). Amsterdam: Swets & Zeitlinger

Svebak, S., & Apter, M. J. (1987). Laughter: An empirical test of some reversal theory hypotheses. *Scandinavian Journal of Psychology, 28*, 189–198.

Svebak, S., & Stoyva, J. (1980). High arousal can be pleasant and exciting: The theory of psychological reversals. *Biofeedback and Self-Regulation, 5*, 439–444.

Ursin, H., Endresen, I. M., & Ursin, G. (1988). Psychological factors and self-reports of muscle pain. *European Journal of Applied Physiology, 52*, 282–290.

Wyer, R. S., & Collins, J. E. (1992) A theory of humor elicitation. *Psychological Review, 99*, 663–688.

Yovetich, N. A., Dale, J. A., & Hudak, M. A. (1990). Benefits of humor in reduction of threat-induced anxiety. *Psychological Reports, 66*, 51–58.

15

Stress, Exercise, and Sport

John H. Kerr

This chapter outlines the important role that exercise and sport can play in dealing with stress-related problems and psychological health and well-being. Although these activities may not be suitable for everyone, the author points out that, for some, there are at least two ways in which exercise and sport may be effective as stress management techniques. For some individuals experiencing tension-stress, the use of exercise and sport, as a means of modulating arousal, as a means of reversal induction, or as both may prove effective. The results of recent empirical research are used to illustrate how these coping strategies might work as part of the reversal theory approach to stress management. Other later parts of the chapter draw attention to the need to match exercise and sports activities with metamotivational style (dominance) and underline how engaging in exercise and sport activities may be counterproductive for some people.

In the majority of the economically well-developed countries, health, occupational, and counseling psychologists have realized that exercise participation can play a role in the maintenance of psychological health (see, e.g., Kerr, Cox, & Griffiths, 1996). This is especially true for those members of these groups who are involved in the prevention and management of stress. Of late, exercise is frequently being included with other, longer established stress management interventions (e.g., meditation, progressive relaxation) as a possible stress management intervention (see, e.g., Ivancevich, Matteson, Freedman, & Phillips, 1990).

Other health care providers are promoting physical exercise as a critical component in the development and maintenance of a healthy lifestyle. Health clinics and other facilities often promote physical activity and exercise through booklets and self-help kits, and some health care professionals offer physical activity counseling (Pender, Sallis, Long, & Calfas, 1994). Mirroring this trend in the health professions are similar initiatives by schools (especially in physical education curricula), neighborhood community organizations, businesses and other organizations, and private health facilities, spas, and clubs (King, 1994). Rather than being concerned with psychological health, often the primary concern of these different groups has been with the promotion of physical activity and exercise as protection against cardiovascular diseases, especially coronary heart disease, obesity, and other physical problems arising from nonactive lifestyles.

Physical and psychological health are, of course, related and any possible benefits from exercise participation are not likely to accrue in any isolated or exclusive manner. Improvements in physical health are likely to positively influence psychological health and vice versa. For example, people who take up some form of physical exercise to reduce their risk of coronary heart disease may also find that, after a period of time, their affective well-being is also improved. Consequently, dividing human health into physical and psychological components is a rather artificial exercise. However, to address the potential of exercise and sports participation for stress management in the limited space of this chapter, this regrettable but expedient division is made here.

EXERCISE, SPORT, AND STRESS MANAGEMENT

In terms of the tension-stress, which arises in the telic and paratelic states as a result of a mismatch in preferred and actual levels of arousal (see Chapter 2), there would appear to be two ways in which exercise may be effective as a stress management technique (Kerr, 1993). The first of these is concerned with arousal modulation. With regard to paratelic tension-stress and its associated feelings of boredom, going for a run, bike ride, or swim could well increase felt arousal levels and dissipate low arousal and the unpleasant boredom that were the source of tension-stress. Not only would arousal levels be increased during the period of exercise, but they would also be likely to remain at elevated levels for some time postexercise (e.g., Thayer, 1987; Thayer, Peters, Takahashi, & Birkhead-Flight, 1993). Consider also telic tension-stress. In this case, exercise participation would initially do little to decrease the unpleasantly high levels of arousal causing the telic tension-stress. However, it is often reported by regular exercisers and sports participants that they do experience a low arousal state, not immediately, but some time after exercise, characterized by a pleasantly tired feeling in their bodies (e.g., Johnsgard, 1989). Both telic and paratelic tension-stress result from the individual experiencing either too low or too high levels of felt arousal. Exercise participation and the resultant arousal modulation can be thought of as a form of effort-stress that assists the individual in coping (see Figure 1). In this way, exercise or sports participation may prove useful as a stress management intervention for those who suffer from paratelic or telic tension-stress.

The second way in which exercise may be effective as a stress management

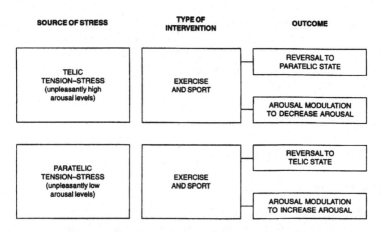

Figure 1   Tension-stress, intervention, and outcomes.

technique derives from the possibility of using exercise activities to evoke reversals (Kerr, 1993). A person experiencing telic or paratelic tension-stress may,
by evoking a reversal to the appropriate opposite metamotivational state, bring
about a reinterpretation of the unpleasant (too low or too high) levels of arousal
and provide some release from the effects of stress (see Figure 1). Taking part
in exercise and sports activities may be an effective way of inducing reversals.
For example, someone may be experiencing telic tension-stress in the form of
anxiety. That person may, by joining colleagues for a game of lunchtime volley-
ball or basketball, evoke a reversal to the paratelic state where his or her unpleasantly high levels of arousal would be experienced as excitement and interest as the play developed. Even if this period in the paratelic state was relatively
short-lived, it would still serve to dissipate some of the immediate effects of
tension-stress and contribute to a more balanced overall metamotivational pattern in the longer term.

For the person experiencing paratelic tension-stress, participation in sports
or exercise activities could evoke a reversal in the opposite direction to the telic
state, where low levels of arousal would be experienced as pleasant relaxation.
However, this stress management strategy is less straightforward than the telic-
to-paratelic reversal strategy. As has been mentioned above, taking part in many
sports and exercise activities tends to increase arousal levels; individuals experiencing paratelic tension-stress should therefore choose activities such as archery,
pistol shooting, Tai Chi, or yoga, which require relaxed concentration and in
which participation does not markedly increase arousal levels. These types of
activities may be suitable for easing the effects of paratelic tension-stress if they
can be made goal-oriented and serious enough to prompt a reversal to the telic
state (see Figure 1).

Keep in mind, however, that the success of these possible sport and
exercise stress management strategies is dependant on the experience of the

individual. For example, sport and exercise (especially sport) can be fun, but it is all too easy for them (especially exercise) to become a chore and a threat. In this way these activities may add to stress rather than help to relieve it. Published research results, generated within a specifically reversal theory framework, have provided evidence that supports the differing roles that sports and exercise activities can play in stress management. This evidence is summarized in the following sections.

REVERSAL THEORY RESEARCH EVIDENCE

Arousal Modulation

Kerr and Vlaswinkel (1993) carried out a two-part field study on male and female regular exercisers to monitor possible changes in their psychological mood and metamotivational states induced by running. The first of these field studies focussed on participants ($N = 32$) in a 7-week program of varied and increasingly demanding running aimed at improving physical fitness. The Telic State Measure (TSM; Svebak & Murgatroyd, 1985) and the Stress Arousal Checklist (SACL; Mackay, Cox, Burrows, & Lazzerini, 1978) were used to measure metamotivational state and aspects of stress and arousal before and after running sessions. The TSM and SACL are short self-report measures that provide indications of (a) whether the telic or paratelic state is operative, (b) levels of preferred and felt arousal, and (c) the level of stress experienced in any situation.

The results of this study indicated that both men and women experienced significant increases in self-reported arousal scores (both felt and preferred arousal) before and after running (see Figures 2A and 2B). For millions of people who play sports or take part in most exercise activities, to state that participation increases levels of arousal is hardly earth-shattering news. For them, this is self-evident. What is of interest here is that the increases in self-reported arousal were accompanied by low levels of stress. Stress levels did increase significantly over the 7 weeks as a consequence of the increasing demands of the running program, but did not increase significantly pre- to postrunning, and overall mean scores remained low. Also, arousal discrepancy scores (a reflection of any mismatch between felt and preferred arousal level) decreased significantly pre- to postrunning. All of this suggests that these regular exercisers experienced arousal increases in a pleasant way (as excitement), providing support for the arousal modulation stress management strategy for dealing with paratelic tension-stress (boredom), outlined above. Similar results were obtained with respect to self-reported arousal in the second part of the study, which used the same instruments, pre- and postrunning, with a different group of 67 regularly exercising male and female participants. Male participants ran 6.6 km and female participants ran 5.0 km at their own pace on trails through natural parkland. Again, in this case the significant increases in self-reported arousal were

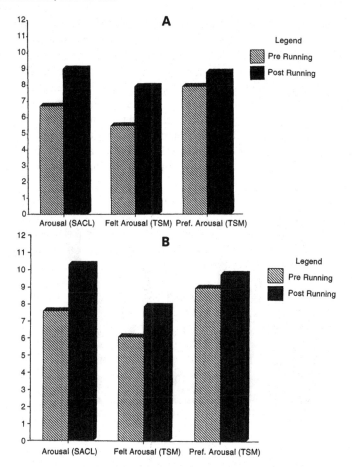

Figure 2 Male participants' (A) and female participants (B) pre- and postrunning mean arousal scores in Study 1. The x-axes show the three SACL–TSM arousal items; y-axes show participants' mean scores on these three items pre- and postrunning. SACL = Stress Arousal Checklist; TSM = Telic State Measure.

not accompanied by significant increases in stress. For this second group of regular runners, the exercise-induced increases in arousal were also experienced as pleasant.

Inducing Reversals

In this second part of the field study (Kerr & Vlaswinkel, 1993), participants were also asked to make color choices (light blue or red) at regular intervals as they ran. The choice of either of these colors at any one time has been shown to be statistically linked to levels of preferred arousal (Walters, Apter, & Svebak, 1982). Specifically, light blue was found to be associated with a preference for low arousal and red with a preference for high arousal. In turn, these colors and the appropriate level of preferred arousal have been shown to be a generally reliable indicator of metamotivational state (light blue for telic, red for paratelic). This allowed ongoing changes in metamotivational state to be monitored during the run. The results showed that the majority of male and female runners preferred lower levels of arousal during the early stages of the run, but during the later stages the majority of participants changed to a preference for high arousal (see Figures 3A and 3B). Thus, it would appear that the change in preference for arousal (through color choice) was indicative of an increasing number of reversals from the telic to the paratelic state as the run progressed. This result

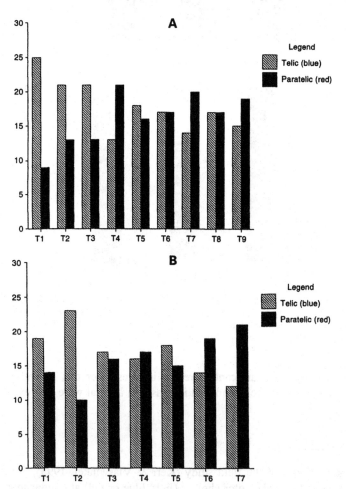

Figure 3 Male participants' (A) and female participants' (B) color choices. The x-axes show the nine times during the run when participants made a color choice (blue = telic, red = paratelic); y-axes show the numbers of participants in the telic and paratelic state at these times.

provides support for the reversal-evoking stress management strategy for dealing with telic tension-stress described earlier.

These two parts of the study are complementary in that they show how running can produce pleasant paratelic high arousal (low tension-stress) in both cases, in Study 1 by increasing arousal in people already in the paratelic state and in Study 2 by both increasing arousal and inducing a reversal to the paratelic state in people who started out in the telic state.

Examination of individual color choice profiles did indicate some variation in the color choice patterns at an individual level, suggesting that although group data indicated a general pattern of reversals from the telic to the paratelic state, not all individuals followed this general trend. In the light of reversal theory, a phenomenologically based theory, this is not surprising. More important, it also serves to demonstrate that running, as a stress management intervention, may be effective in inducing reversals in some individuals but not in others. This is also true of the effectiveness of other stress management interventions (see, e.g., Heide & Borkevec, 1983).

The assertion (Kerr, 1993) that participation in sport may allow people to induce reversals between metamotivational states (particularly the telic and paratelic states) was tested in a different setting. The participants in the study (Kerr & Vlaswinkel, 1995) were 42 postgraduate students enrolled in a very intensive international MBA program. Apart from their work commitments, these students had the opportunity to take part voluntarily in a physical education sports activity on 1 day per week. Groups of participants ($n = 26$) and nonparticipants ($n = 16$) were self-selecting (random allocation of participants to experimental groups was not possible); therefore, a quasi-experimental research design (Cook & Campbell, 1979) was used. Verbal reports from participants who did not take part in the sports activity indicated that they spent the time allocated for sport working. The TSM and the SACL were again used to measure metamotivational state and aspects of stress and arousal on five occasions throughout the day; at the beginning and end of the participants' morning lecture (9:00 a.m. & 12:15 p.m.), just before and immediately after the sport session (1:30 p.m. & 2:15 p.m.), and at the end of the participants' last scheduled lecture (5:00 p.m.). Participants also completed the Telic Dominance Scale (Murgatroyd, Rushton, Apter, & Ray, 1978) on an occasion before the day of the study to ensure that differences in mood response were not a result of group differences in telic dominance. Data analysis confirmed this, and a number of other interesting findings were obtained.

Using the serious—playful Item 1 of the TSM as an indicator of operative state, significantly more participants in the sport group than in the nonsport group were in the paratelic state just after the sport session. At the other four times of measurement, there were no important differences between groups. The pattern of scores on this same item over the day also revealed a significant difference in scores between sport participants and nonsport participants (see Figures 4A and 4B). Scores were similar until just before the sport session

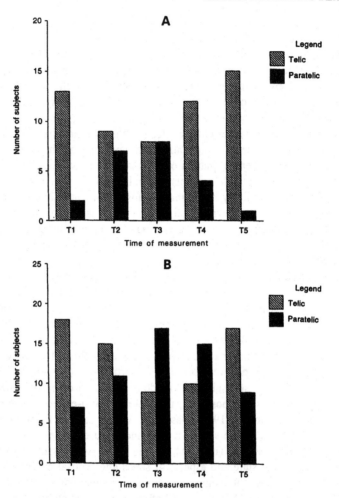

Figure 4 Incidences of telic and paratelic states in the sport group (A) and nonsport group (B) over the day. The x-axes show the five times measurement; y-axes show the numbers of participants in the telic and paratelic states at these times.

where the serious scores of the sports group decreased and those of the nonsport group increased. This pattern continued for the nonsport group, who became increasingly more serious during the afternoon. Sport participants did become more serious after the sport session, but did not achieve the level of the nonsport participants (see Figure 5). A significant main effect on TSM serious–playful scores showed that these participants were less serious, both before and after the session, than nonsport participants. These results provide some evidence that participating in a playful sports session during an otherwise intensive day of (telic-oriented) work activities is likely to induce a reversal to the paratelic state. Although in this case it is possible that a number of sport group participants

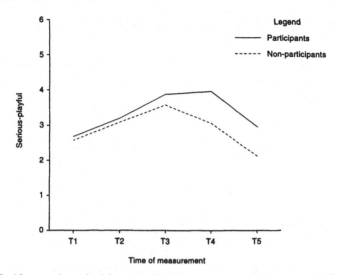

Figure 5 Mean serious-playful scores for the sport and nonsport groups. The x-axis shows the five times of measurement; y-axis shows the sport and nonsport groups' mean serious–playful scores at these times.

may have reversed back to the telic state on resuming their studies, some time was spent in the paratelic state, thus contributing to their general mental health.

Generally, stress levels were not high, but a significant interaction effect was found for SACL stress scores, which indicated that the sport group reported higher SACL stress levels before and lower SACL stress levels after the sport session than did nonsport participants. This finding suggests that the prospect of participating in physically demanding sport activities may initially increase stress levels to some extent, but participation in a "time out" activity, such as sport, may subsequently reduce stress levels (Morgan, 1987). Sport and exercise may therefore perform what Apter (1990, p. 52) called a "mental hygiene service" for those who take advantage of it.

Reversal theory–based research on the potential of exercise and sport for stress management is in its early stages. The results of the two studies described above do indicate that the claims made about modulation of arousal levels and the inducement of reversals are not without substance. These results are important when considered alongside the results of other research studies that have confirmed the role that exercise can play in preventing or moderating the effects of stress (e.g., Long & Haney, 1988; Moses, Steptoe, Mathews, & Edwards, 1989; Norris, Carroll, & Cochrane, 1992). There is a need, however, for further research that addresses the other stress management strategies proposed in this chapter. In particular, the role of low arousal in relaxed concentration activities like archery and Tai Chi in coping with paratelic tension-stress and the mechanisms involved in longer term postexercise decreases in arousal for helping with telic tension-stress need to be explored.

MATCHING SPORTS AND EXERCISE ACTIVITIES
WITH MOTIVATIONAL STYLE

Some observers of public attitudes to, and trends in, exercise participation and adherence (e.g., Dishman, 1994, p. VII) have conceded that the exercise promotion programs of the 1980s have been largely unsuccessful in increasing participation and that attempts to explain why well-intentioned people remain inactive or return to inactivity even after periods of successful exercise have also failed. Even though modest increases in physical activity may result from exercise interventions, many are short-lived, without permanent changes and sustained activity.

Often people not accustomed to exercising or playing sports begin to do so because a particular activity is "in" at a particular time. Over recent years, there have been fads or crazes for jogging, in-line skating, working out with weights, treadmill running and stair climbing, aerobic dancing, mountain biking, swimming, and other types of activities. People try the latest exercise fad, and some find it enjoyable and continue to participate, whereas others, probably the majority, stop after a period and perhaps move on to the next in activity. Among those who drop out, interest is often, at best, transitory. One possible reason why adherence to sports and exercise is poor and drop-out rates are high is that people fail to choose to take part in activities that match their motivational style (i.e., dominance).

A number of reversal theory research studies (Kerr, 1991; Kerr & Svebak, 1989; Svebak & Kerr, 1989) have found important links between the types of sports and exercise activities that people prefer and participate in and individual motivational style. For example, sports involving repetitive rhythmical movements and high levels of endurance appear to be suited to telic-dominant individuals, and sports requiring quick reactions and sudden explosive movements, such as baseball or cricket, appear to be suited to paratelic-dominant individuals (Svebak & Kerr, 1989). Conversely, sports that involve an element of physical risk such as surfing, parachuting, or motor sports are performed by individuals who exhibit paratelic dominance. Other, safer sports, like long-distance running and weight training are performed by telic-dominant individuals (e.g., Kerr, 1991; Kerr & Svebak, 1989; Summers & Stewart, 1993). The consequence of this is that, if a paratelic-dominant individual takes up jogging, he or she is unlikely to find it satisfying in terms of motivational needs. In other words, the paratelic-dominant person experiencing paratelic tension-stress is unlikely to find jogging or any other endurance sport useful as a stress management technique. What they are likely to find effective in managing stress is a sport characterized by explosive movements and action or risk-taking with which they can satisfy their tendency for arousal seeking and experience high levels of arousal as pleasant excitement. Conversely, the telic-dominant person should avoid these latter sports and take part in endurance-type and safer sports and exercise activities. This is especially true for the telic-dominant person experiencing telic tension-stress. For them, effective stress management through exercise and sports is more likely through participation in sports and exercise activities that suit their arousal-avoiding motivational style.

In reversal theory terms, a necessary requirement for the maintenance of sound psychological health is that the individual be able to experience the full range of metamotivational states on a relatively frequent basis. As a result, frequent reversals between different metamotivational states are a necessary part of this process. Murgatroyd and Apter (1984, 1986), however, have identified two basic types of reversal disturbances that, if they endure over time, are likely to result in clinical problems for the individual concerned. These are inappropriate reversal and reversal inhibition (see, e.g., Murgatroyd & Apter, 1984, 1986). It has been argued above that sport and exercise may assist in the reversal process, and similar arguments hold true for people with clinical problems arising from reversal process disturbances. For example, reversal inhibition occurs when person is trapped in one particular metamotivational state and is unable to reverse easily and frequently in a healthy way to the opposite state. These circumstances often apply to the telic-dominant person experiencing prolonged periods of unpleasantly high arousal in the telic state (telic tension-stress), which may then manifest itself, for example, as chronic anxiety. For this person, sport, because of its playful nature, may be especially effective in inducing the paratelic state and relieving stress to some degree. However, for some individuals experiencing reversal inhibition, engaging in exercise and sport may be counterproductive. There is a possibility that, rather than acting to evoke the paratelic state, the sport and exercise activity (especially the latter) may be approached in the same manner as other activities and become an added stressor, thus trapping the individual further in the telic state and exacerbating the existing problem. This may be especially true for exercise activities that are attractive to telic-dominant individuals and that can easily take on a telic orientation with some individuals who become obsessional about participation and the pursuit of exercise goals. Consequently, as with all stress management strategies, some caution is required in recommending particular interventions, and subsequent evaluation of their effectiveness is a necessity.

CONCLUSION

There are very few, if any, other theoretical perspectives on the concept of stress that advocate putting yourself under more stress to relieve the symptoms of stress. That apparently contradictory suggestion is precisely what reversal theory advocates when exercise and sports activities are recommended for use as coping mechanisms for counteracting some forms of stress. Apter (1990) captured the essence of this approach in a nutshell,

> It is a widespread assumption these days that behaviors which display competitiveness, time urgency, hostility and aggression, and experiences which involve con-

frontation and threat, are stressful and likely to be damaging to the health of those who indulge in them. And yet these kinds of behaviors and experiences are exactly what sport is all about. A game without confrontation would be no game at all. A contest with no competition would be no contest. It would therefore seem to follow that engaging in sport would be the worst thing anyone could do. . . . And yet clearly sport is not stressful in this sense. (p. 52)

As with topics in other areas of psychology, reversal theory has challenged conventional approaches to the study of stress (see Chapter 2). The ideas put forward in this chapter with regard to exercise and sport may be of use to those care professionals from health, counseling, and exercise psychology mentioned earlier. To date, they have experienced some difficulty in finding a satisfactory theoretical basis for their work. Reversal theory provides them with an opportunity to locate exercise and sport-based therapy within an innovative, but comprehensive, theoretical structure. By doing so, justification for the inclusion of these activities in stress interventions aimed at coping with different forms of stress can be strengthened considerably. The task for reversal theorists, or at least those reversal theorists interested in exercise and sport, is to continue with their investigations and further establish the promising beginning the reversal theory approach to stress and stress management has made thus far.

REFERENCES

Apter, M. J. (1990). Sport and mental health: A new psychological perspective. In G. P. H. Hermans & W. L. Mosterd (Eds.), *Sports, medicine and health* (Excerpta Medica International Congress Series, pp. 47–56). Amsterdam: Elsevier.

Cook, T. D., & Campbell, D. T. (1979). *Quasi-experimentation: Design and analysis for field settings.* Boston: Houghton Mifflin .

Dishman, R. K. (1994). *Advances in exercise adherence.* Champaign, IL: Human Kinetics.

Heide, F. J., & Borkevec, T. D. (1983). Relaxation and induced anxiety-paradoxical anxiety enhancement due to relaxation training. *Journal of Consulting and Clinical Psychology, 51,* 171–182.

Ivancevich, J. M., Matteson, M. T., Freedman, S. M., & Phillips, J. S. (1990). Worksite stress management interventions. *American Psychologist, 45,* 252–261.

Johnsgard, K. W. (1989). *The exercise prescription for depression and anxiety.* New York: Plenum Press.

Kerr, J. H. (1991). Arousal-seeking in risk sport participants. *Personality and Individual Differences, 12,* 613–616.

Kerr, J. H. (1993). Employee exercise breaks: Opportunities for reversal. In J. H. Kerr, S. Murgatroyd, & M. J. Apter (Eds.), *Advances in reversal theory* (pp. 247–256). Amsterdam: Swets & Zeitlinger.

Kerr, J. H., Cox, T., & Griffiths, A. (1995). *Workplace health: Employee fitness and exercise.* London: Taylor & Francis.

Kerr, J. H., & Svebak, S. (1989). Motivational aspects of preference for and participation in risk sports. *Personality and Individual Differences, 10,* 797–800.

Kerr, J. H., & Vlaswinkel, E. H. (1993). Self-reported mood and running under natural conditions. *Work & Stress, 7,* 161–177.

Kerr, J. H., & Vlaswinkel, E. H. (1995). Sport participation at work: An aid to stress management? *International Journal of Stress Management, 2,* 87–96.

King, A. C. (1994). Clinical and community interventions to promote and support physical activity participation. In R. K. Dishman (Ed.), *Advances in exercise adherence*. Champaign, IL: Human Kinetics.

Long, B. C., & Haney, C. J. (1988). Coping strategies for working women: Aerobic exercise and relaxation interventions. *Behavior Therapy, 19,* 75–83.

Mackay, C. J., Cox, T., Burrows, G., & Lazzerini, A. J. (1978). An inventory for the measurement of self reported stress and arousal. *British Journal of Social and Clinical Psychology, 17,* 283–284.

Morgan, W. P. (1987). Reduction of state anxiety following acute physical activity. In W. P. Morgan & S. E. Goldstein (Eds.), *Exercise and mental health* (pp. 105–115). Washington: Hemisphere.

Moses, J., Steptoe, A., Mathews, A., & Edwards, S. (1989). The effects of exercise training on mental well-being in the normal population: A controlled study. *Journal of Psychosomatic Research, 33,* 47–61.

Murgatroyd, S., & Apter, M. J. (1984). Eclectic psychotherapy: A structural-phenomenological approach. In W. Dryden (Ed.), *Individual psychotherapy in Britain* (pp. 392–414). London: Harper & Row.

Murgatroyd, S., & Apter, M. J. (1986). A structural-phenomenological approach to eclectic psychotherapy. In J. Norcross (Ed.), *Handbook of eclectic psychotherapy* (pp. 260–280). New York: Brunner/Mazel.

Murgatroyd, S., Rushton, C., Apter, M. J., & Ray, C. (1978). The development of the Telic Dominance Scale. *Journal of Personality Assessment, 42,* 519–522.

Norris, R., Carroll, D., & Cochrane, R. (1992). The effects of physical activity and exercise training on psychological stress and well-being in an adolescent population. *Journal of Psychosomatic Research, 36,* 55–65.

Pender, N. J., Sallis, J. F., Long, B. J., & Calfas, K. J. (1994). Health-care provider counseling to promote physical activity. In R. K. Dishman (Ed.), *Advances in exercise adherence* (pp. 213–235). Champaign, IL: Human Kinetics.

Summers, J., & Stewart, E. (1993, June). *The arousal-performance relationship: Examining differing conceptions.* Paper presented at the 8th World Congress in Sport Psychology, Lisbon, Portugal.

Svebak, S., & Kerr, J. H. (1989). The role of impulsivity in preference for sports. *Personality and Individual Differences, 10,* 51–58.

Svebak, S., & Murgatroyd, S. (1985). Metamotivational dominance: A multimethod validation of reversal theory constructs. *Journal of Personality and Social Psychology, 48,* 107–116.

Thayer, R. E. (1987). Energy, tiredness, and tension effects of a sugar snack versus moderate exercise. *Journal of Personality and Social Psychology, 52,* 119–125.

Thayer, R. E., Peters, D. P., Takahashi, P. J., & Birkhead-Flight, A. M. (1993). Mood and behavior (smoking and sugar snacking) following moderate exercise: A partial test of self-regulation theory. *Personality and Individual Differences, 14,* 97–104.

Walters, J. M., Apter, M. J., & Svebak, S. (1982). Color preference, arousal and the theory of psychological reversals. *Motivation and Emotion, 6,* 193–215.

16

Stress in the Workplace: Causes and Treatments

David Fontana and Lucilia Valente

The models proposed by reversal theory are potentially of great help in the identification of the organizational and personal factors that prompt stress in working life. The theory also provides researchers with an interactive model that helps illuminate the manner in which organizations and individuals create stress-promoting variables through a mismatch between organizational climate and individual metamotivational modes. Arising from an understanding of these variables are a number of practical strategies for use within stress management workshops. The chapter presents this interactive model in the context of the telic–paratelic, mastery–sympathy, negativistic–conformist, and autic–alloic dimensions and outlines these practical strategies.

Not only have the effects of stress—both psychological and physiological—been widely investigated over the years (e.g., Benson & Klipper, 1975; Fontana, 1989; Selye, 1978), but so have its antecedents and moderators. Of particular psychological interest have been the studies of life events most likely to produce stress (Holmes & Rahe, 1967), together with the personality variables that may render individuals most susceptible to stress-inducing pressures. Among these personality variables are locus of control (Lefcourt, Miller, Ware, & Sherk, 1981); inadequate sense of humor (Lefcourt & Martin, 1986); and extraversion, neuroticism, and psychoticism (Fontana & Abouserie, 1993), which may make individuals more vulnerable to these and other experiences. However, because the causes of stress are both person-specific and situation-specific, any model capable of discriminating stress-vulnerable individuals must of necessity be an interactive one, linking particular situations to particular participants.

The reversal theory model of stress (see, e.g., Apter & Svebak, 1989; Baker,

1988; and Chapter 2) goes further than many other models in that it is able usefully to address the relationship between the organizational climate in the workplace and the individual's reactions to this climate. In consequence, it has the potential to act in an interactive capacity, and thus to prompt appropriate change at both institutional and personal levels.

STRESS SUSCEPTIBILITY

The psychologically healthy person is defined by Murgatroyd and Apter (1984, 1986) as someone who, among other things, is "inherently inconsistent"—that is, as someone who can reverse readily, even in the face of relatively stable outer situations, between the metamotivational modes at opposite ends of the various dimensions identified by reversal theory. When applied to stress, such a definition implies that an inability to reverse as appropriate in the face of potentially stress-promoting variables (whether situational or personal) may be a major factor in vulnerability to stress.

All this is consistent with earlier work by Apter and one of the present authors (e.g., Fontana, 1981) that established that the obsessional personality shows rigid location in the telic mode (telic dominance) and thus lacks the facility to experience the reversals into the paratelic mode that in certain circumstances are of potential help as stress-coping mechanisms. It also accords with work by Svebak (1988) that links the Type A personality with dominance, respectively, in the arousal-avoiding, negativistic, autocentric, and mastery metamotivational modes identified by reversal theory. Equally important, it is consistent with findings by Martin, Kuiper, and Olinger (1988) that link telic dominance with an aversive and deleterious response to stressors and link paratelic dominance with a boredom response in the absence—at least at a mild level—of such stressors.

REVERSAL THEORY PROVIDES AN INTERACTIVE MODEL OF STRESS VULNERABILITY

Reversal theory, then, leads to the proposal that vulnerability to stress may be more prevalent among those unable to reverse readily and appropriately out of their dominant mode (reversal-inhibited individuals). The question then arises for this interactive reversal theory model of stress vulnerability as to the person-specific workplace situations in which this inability will be potentially most harmful. Once again, reversal theory provides a clear range of clues. One can list the recognizable situations, or types of corporate culture or organizational climate suggested by these clues, together with the functional metamotivational modes of those likely to be more stress-prone when confronted by them. In other words, where there is a mismatch between climate and ongoing mode, tension-stress (as defined in Chapter 2) is likely to be a consequence, possibly leading to effort-stress. For example, tension-stress in the form of anxiety might occur in Case A in the list below and in the form of boredom in Case B, and then effort-stress would arise in the event of an effortful attempt by the individual concerned to overcome the effect of these mismatches. The following list, then, documents all the possible kinds of person–organization mismatches that can occur at the metamotivational level.

Telic–Paratelic Dimension

Organizational climate   Stress-prone mode

A. Unstructured and open-ended, with   Telic
elements of ambiguity; rewards given
unpredictably and for feeling-related behaviors.

B. Highly convergent and goal-directed; rewards   Paratelic
given for clearly defined and recognizable
task-related behaviors.

Negativistic–Conformist Dimension

Organizational climate   Stress-prone mode

C. Rule-governed and specific; rewards given   Negativistic
for obedience and subordination.

D. Confrontative and individualistic; rewards   Conformist
given for cussedness and persistence.

Mastery–Sympathy Dimension

Organizational climate   Stress-prone mode

E. Supportive, responsive, or democratic;   Mastery
rewards given for people-centered behaviors.

F. Authoritarian and hierarchical; rewards   Sympathy
given for tough-minded behaviors.

Autic–Alloic Dimension

Organizational climate   Stress-prone mode

G. Encourages autonomy, rewards given for   Alloic
personal excellence.

H. Encourages teamwork and identification with   Autic
the organization; rewards given for selflessness.

Individuals may, of course, manifest elements of each of the above four modes at different times, and workplace situations may include more than one of the listed situations. Thus, the interactive model may in due course need to be broadened to take account of possible multiple interactions. Also, individuals may differ in terms of how vulnerable to tension- and effort-stress they are in different modes. As an initial statement of the model, however, the above demonstrates the power of reversal theory to link situation to subject in a way not readily apparent in other psychological theories of motivation. Further, it not only offers theoretical integrity, it provides the basis for clear guidance on the forms that therapeutic intervention with stress-vulnerable individuals might best take, and these are returned to in due course.

RELEVANCE FOR DOMESTIC STRESS

The emphasis of this chapter is on stress in occupational life. However, it is likely that the model may also have some relevance for stress in home life. At face value, it is reasonable to propose that within domestic relationships and home management, reversal-inhibited individuals may encounter stress when confronted with domestic versions of the situations just described. The above model cannot of course account for all domestic stress. There will be many other factors at work, and other reasons for the domestic incompatibility and discord that lead to stress (not least of them a failure to agree on when one partner as opposed to the other should be required to reverse). Both occupational and domestic life are significantly about relationships, however, and Apter (e.g., Apter, 1982) has already identified a lack of harmony between the preferred metamotivational modes of individuals as a potent cause of problems both in relationships between adults and in those between adults and children.

STRESS-MANAGEMENT TECHNIQUES DERIVED
FROM REVERSAL THEORY

It has been found that when using the reversal theory model in individual counseling or in stress management workshops, it is important to establish at the outset the situation or situations within which clients have to conduct their working lives. The second step is to arrive at an assessment of their dominant metamotivational modes and the facility with which they can reverse appropriately between modes, and to identify where mismatches between organizational climate and individuals occur. The third step is to examine how such mismatches can best be resolved in reversal theory terms. These three steps can be tackled as follows.

Step 1: Dominant Metamotivational Modes Within
the Occupational Environment

It is likely that, in due course, standardized psychometric instruments will be developed that will enable researchers and therapists to categorize institutions and their organizational climates in terms of dominant metamotivational modes, much as it is currently possible to categorize people in this way. Institutions are human creations and reflect— and in turn react with and influence— the preferred modes of those who manage them, whether these modes are self-determined or shaped by market and economic forces.

Until standardized instruments are available for measuring organizational climate in reversal theory terms, the most satisfactory approach at workshop level is to provide participants with simple checklists that help them identify the predominant mode (or modes) of the institutions in which they are employed. The exercise carries its own validity in that it is the individual's perception of his or her institution, whether properly objective or not, that is of most importance.

The items that make up these checklists can be selected by workshop participants themselves, working in small groups with each group requested to decide on the relevant variables in a specific area of the organizational climate (e.g., relationships with superiors, task demands, recognition and reinforcement, relationships with colleagues, decision-making processes, channels of communication, relationships with clients). An alternative is to take suitable items from the measuring instruments now available within reversal theory for assessing individual metamotivational modes (mentioned under Step 2) and reword them into a format suitable for the assessment of institutions rather than persons. Whichever approach is used, however, the aim of the checklist is to allow participants to build up a comprehensive picture of the dominant metamotivational modes that appear to characterize the climate of the institution within which they work.

To avoid the induction of mental set when tackling Step 2, it is better not to assign overall characterizations to institutions on the basis of the work done in Step 1 until this second step is completed.

Step 2: Dominant Metamotivational Modes Within Individuals

Psychometric scales for assessing telic–paratelic dominance (e.g., the Telic Dominance Scale [Murgatroyd, Rushton, Apter, & Ray, 1978], and the Paratelic Dominance Scale [Cook & Gerkovich, 1993]) and for assessing negativism–conformity (the Negativism Dominance Scale; McDermott, 1988) are now available (see Apter, 1989, for a full discussion). In addition, a psychometric instrument known as the Motivational Style Profile is currently being developed by Apter and others to measure all the dominances postulated by reversal theory and will thus, among other things, provide assessments of the mastery–sympathy and autic–alloic dimensions (Apter & Apter-Desselles, 1993).

The use of such psychometric instruments, together with the discussion to which this gives rise, provides workshop participants with an initiation into reversal theory at the functional level, and it is at this point that the material generated in Step 1 can now be explored in reversal theory terms. As a consequence, individuals gain an awareness both of their own metamotivational modes and of the climate prevailing within the institutions for which they work, and in this way mismatches between the two can be identified, explored, and discussed.

Workshop participants can also be also be prompted during Step 2 to explore the ease with which they can reverse between the modes they have identified in themselves. As indicated at the outset of the chapter, it is reversal inhibition, the inability to reverse readily and appropriately between modes, that is considered by reversal theory to be a major cause of psychological problems, rather than mode dominance itself. As is clear from the first two chapters of this book, reversal theory differs from trait-based theories of personality and from the theory of homeostasis in that it suggests that psychological health requires the ability to reverse between opposite modes of psychological functioning rather than staying located in one or the other or remaining in equilibrium between them. Thus, an individual is not regarded as showing psychological malaise because he or she is, for example, telic-dominant or paratelic-dominant, but because he or she is unable to reverse from the dominant mode into its opposite on those occasions when it would be most appropriate to do so.

Scores on the measuring instruments mentioned above provide some insight into the ease with which reversals can take place for a given participant. Scores toward the extreme of any one mode suggest, ipso facto, that reversal into its opposite may be more difficult or may produce feelings of discomfort. Introspection can, however, also be helpful in relation to each pair of states. After examining and discussing the metamotivational profile revealed by the instruments, a participant is able to review personal experience and offer conclusions as to whether or not reversal comes easily to him or her.

Of course, even where reversal from the dominant mode into its alternative for each pair of states can be effected as required, an individual may develop negative attitudes toward the organization if he or she has to stay indefinitely in his or her nondominant mode for a given pair. The individual's dominant mode may well be the one that he or she prefers, and it is often right and reasonable that the individual will wish to work within an occupational environment that favors this preferred mode.

After Steps 1 and 2 have been completed, participants have an awareness of the factors in their organizational climate, together with the factors in themselves, that are contributing to their unacceptable levels of occupational stress. As in any psychological exercise that leads to greater self- and self–other understanding, this awareness per se can have a liberating effect on many individuals (Apter & Smith, 1979). Occupational stress is now seen by them as something that is comprehensible, and therefore amenable to coping strategies. This allows participants to move with some confidence to Step 3.

Step 3: The Resolution of Mismatches Between Institutional and Personal Metamotivational Modes

There are three major coping strategies that emerge in Step 3. These are (a) changes in the dominant organizational climate, initiated by institutions; (b) changes in the dominant metamotivational modes, initiated by individuals; and (c) decisions on severance and re-employment elsewhere.

Strategy 1 is normally feasible only where the whole of a management team or a sales team are involved in the workshop, and where changes can be made without sacrificing business efficiency or productive capacity. However, where these conditions are met, Strategy 1 can be a highly viable proposition. Discord between members of a management team as a consequence of a mismatch between organizational climate and the metamotivational modes of individuals can sometimes be resolved, and overall operational policies can be revised. It is often only when individuals are brought together in the appropriate environment of an in-house workshop that they become aware of the extent to which current management styles are inappropriate, or are misunderstood by others, or produce mismatches with other styles. It may also only be within the context of such workshops that the negative effects on efficiency and productivity of inappropriate styles become apparent.

Strategy 2 is a viable proposition in all situations where individuals do not suffer from reversal inhibition and where they are able to recognize that reversals are acceptable to their value systems. Once again, it may be that only within the context of a workshop does the need for reversal by individuals into opposite metamotivational modes become apparent. Without a framework within which to examine behavior more precisely, it is often difficult for individuals to recognize the extent to which their own behavior is an actual cause of the stress-related problems with which they feel themselves to be confronted. The workshop not only facilitates such recognition, it also allows individuals to discuss with others the extent to which a reversal in mode is required and the precise circumstances in which it may be most effective. Further, it may even lead to that exploration into the concepts of self and of personal identity that reversal theory also offers (Fontana, 1988).

Strategies for assisting reversal-inhibited individuals to examine the reasons for their inhibitions and to identify possible ways of coping with them are discussed in Murgatroyd and Apter (1984, 1986), but Fontana and Valente (1993) have suggested that role-play and simulation exercises, together with various of the other techniques used in dramatherapy, are of value here. Dramatherapy techniques, by giving participants permission to function in metamotivational modes opposite to those in which they normally operate, can help them recognize and develop hitherto dormant potentialities. There is, of course, a difference between acting out a role in a dramatherapy exercise and actually entering the metamotivational mode that gives rise to natural behaviors consistent with that role; however, experience has shown that role-playing and other dramatherapy techniques can be potent methods of self-discovery and can lead to long-term personal changes that in the authors' view are likely to be linked to changes at the metamotivational level.

It must be stressed, however, that Strategy 3 involves important career choices for which only the individuals concerned can take final responsibility. A range of variables outside those dealt with by reversal theory normally must also be taken into consideration. Discussion within the workshop, however, can help participants, where appropriate, to identify and clarify alternatives to their present occupational situations and to assess the possible consequences of applying for and gaining employment within one or another of these alternatives. Such discussion necessarily involves an examination of the metamotivational modes likely to operate as part of the occupational environment obtaining in these alternatives, or at the very least ways of identifying these states before moving toward firm future career decisions. There is nothing particularly esoteric about this exercise. Reversal theory is simply providing individuals with a useful method of formalizing the way in which they analyze the important, but normally imprecise, variables that are subsumed under the heading of organizational climate. In other words, it provides a framework within which they can make informed decisions about changes they might want to make in their lives.

CONSCIOUSLY CHANGING METAMOTIVATIONAL MODES

Are people able consciously to address and effect changes in their metamotivational modes in the way implied in Step 2? Researchers on reversal theory seem to be currently somewhat ambivalent about this, although Apter continues to argue that reversals themselves are always involuntary in the strictest sense of the term. Apter (1989) referred to a range of psychological factors capable of inducing reversals involuntarily (i.e., contingency, satiation, frustration). He also pointed out, however, that individuals may change mode by consciously bringing about alterations in their environmental conditions, for example, by watching television to induce the paratelic mode, thus deliberately inducing contingent reversals, albeit in an indirect way and by means of involuntary mechanisms. Many, including the present authors, would, however, argue that it is possible that people are able in an important sense to voluntarily change mode directly. Cognitive therapies generally (e.g., Clarkson, 1995) accord the individual a fair degree of direct control over motivation and mood, and the present authors' counseling experience (particularly in dramatherapy) suggests that people can indeed think themselves into a particular role and quickly acquire the metamotivational state to accompany it. This is perhaps still technically involuntary, but it certainly comes close to being voluntary in that the cognitive processes are under voluntary control, no input is required from the environment, and reversal may be accomplished almost instantaneously. The whole thing may be accomplished so effortlessly that there is a sense in which effectively, and for all practical purposes, the process is voluntary.

For present purposes, however, there is no need to pursue this issue further. What is important is that shifts in the organizational climate can incorporate the environmental changes that Apter (1989) recognized are responsible for inducing appropriate reversals and for lessening the risk of inappropriate ones. By introducing these environmental changes, and by increasing the situational awareness of all concerned, changes in contingency variables can facilitate desirable reversals in individuals' metamotivational modes. By the same token, reductions in the risk of frustration can help prevent shifts into unsuitable modes. Through the greater self-knowledge that comes from the workshop experiences outlined in this chapter, individuals may also be helped to recognize those indirect means under their control that can induce reversals (e.g., task-switching, context-changing, and focus-switching).

CONCLUSION

Reversal theory provides a clear conceptual foundation for identifying and dealing with some of the important factors that help generate stress in occupational life. It would be wrong to pretend that the theory, as it stands at present, can cover all aspects of stress in the workplace, but more perhaps than any other psychological theory it does have the power to identify a range of potentially important stress-promoting variables in institutions and in the way in which they interact with individuals. Further, it suggests an approach toward coping with these variables by both managers and employees that can readily be put to practical use within stress management workshops, and in other ways.

REFERENCES

Apter, M. J. (1982). *The experience of motivation: The theory of psychological reversals*. Chichester: Wiley.

Apter, M. J. (1989). *Reversal theory: Motivation, emotion and personality*. London: Routledge.

Apter, M. J., & Apter-Desselles, M. (1993). The personality of the patient: Going beyond the trait concept. *Patient Education and Counseling, 22,* 107–114.

Apter, M. J., & Smith, K. C. P. (1979). Psychological reversals: Some new perspectives on the family and family communication. *Family Therapy, 6,* 89–100.

Apter, M. J., & Svebak, S. (1989). Stress from the reversal theory perspective. In C. D. Spielberger & J. Strelau (Eds.), *Stress and emotion* (Vol. 12, pp. 323–353). New York: McGraw Hill.

Baker, J. (1988). Stress appraisals and coping with everyday hassles. In M. J. Apter, J. H. Kerf, & M. P. Cowles (Eds.), *Progress in reversal theory* (pp. 117–128). Amsterdam: North Holland.

Benson, H., & Klipper, M. Z. (1975). *The relaxation response*. New York: William Morrow.

Clarkson, P. (1995). *The therapeutic relationship*. London: Whurr.

Cook, M., & Gerkovich, M. (1993). The development of a paratelic dominance scale. In J. H. Kerf, S. Murgatroyd, & M. J. Apter (Eds.), *Advances in reversal theory* (pp. 177–188). Amsterdam: Swets & Zeitlinger.

Fontana, D. (1981). Obsessionality and reversal theory. *British Journal of Clinical Psychology, 20,* 229–300.

Fontana, D. (1988). Self-awareness and self-forgetting: Now I see me, now I don't. In M. J.

Apter, J. H. Kerf, & M. P. Cowles (Eds.), *Progress in reversal theory* (pp. 349–357). Amsterdam: North Holland Press.

Fontana, D. (1989). *Managing stress*. London: British Psychological Society/Routledge.

Fontana, D., & Abouserie, R. (1993). Stress levels, gender and personality factors in teachers. *British Journal of Educational Psychology, 63,* 261–270.

Fontana, D., & Valente, L. (1993). Reversal theory, drama and psychological health. In M. J. Apter, S. Murgatroyd, & J. H. Kerf (Eds.), *Advances in reversal theory* (pp. 325–333). Amsterdam: Swets & Zeitlinger

Holmes, T. H., & Rahe, R. H. (1967). The social readjustment rating scale. *Journal of Psychosomatic Research, 11,* 213–218.

Lefcourt, H. M., & Martin, R. A. (1986). *Humor and life stress: Antidote to adversity.* New York: Springer-Verlag.

Lefcourt, H. M., Miller, R. J., Ware, E. E., & Sherk, D. (1981). Locus of control as a modifier of the relationship between stressors and moods. *Journal of Personality and Social Psychology, 45,* 337–369.

Martin, R. A., Kuiper, N. A., & Olinger, L. J. (1988). Telic versus paratelic dominance as a moderation of stress. In M. J. Apter, J. H. Kerr, & M. P. Cowles (Eds.), *Progress in reversal theory* (pp. 107–116). Amsterdam: North Holland Press.

McDermott, M. (1988). Measuring rebelliousness: The development of the Negativism Dominance Scale. In M. J. Apter, J. H. Kerf, & M. P. Cowles, *Progress in reversal theory* (pp. 297–312). Amsterdam: North Holland Press.

Murgatroyd, S., & Apter, M. J. (1984). Eclectic psychotherapy—A structural phenomenological approach. In W. Dryden (Ed.), *Individual psychotherapy in Britain* (pp. 389–414). London: Harper & Row.

Murgatroyd, S., & Apter, M. J. (1986). A structural phenomenological approach to eclectic psychotherapy. In J. C. Norcross (Ed.), *Handbook of eclectic psychotherapy* (pp. 260–280). New York: Brunner/Mazel.

Murgatroyd, S., Rushton, C., Apter, M. J., & Ray, C. (1978). *Journal of Personality Assessment, 42,* 519–528.

Selye, H. (1978). *The stress of life.* New York: McGraw Hill.

Svebak, S. (1988). Personality, stress and cardiovascular risk. In M. J. Apter, J. H. Kerf, & M. P. Cowles (Eds.), *Progress in reversal theory* (pp. 163–172). Amsterdam: North-Holland.

Index

Printed in the United States
by Baker & Taylor Publisher Services